LONG ILLNESS

A PRACTICAL GUIDE
TO SURVIVING,
HEALING, AND THRIVING

MEGHAN JOBSON, MD, PhD, and
JULIET MORGAN, MD

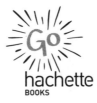

hachette
BOOKS

NEW YORK

Hachette Go, an imprint of Hachette Books
Hachette Book Group
1290 Avenue of the Americas
New York, NY 10104
HachetteGo.com
Facebook.com/HachetteGo
Instagram.com/HachetteGo

First Edition: May 2023

Hachette Books is a division of Hachette Book Group, Inc.
The Hachette Go and Hachette Books name and logos are trademarks of Hachette Book Group, Inc.

The Hachette Speakers Bureau provides a wide range of authors for speaking events.
To find out more, go to hachettespeakersbureau.com or email HachetteSpeakers@hbgusa.com.

Hachette Go books may be purchased in bulk for business, educational, or promotional use. For information, please contact your local bookseller or Hachette Book Group Special Markets Department at: Special.Markets@hbgusa.com.

The publisher is not responsible for websites (or their content) that are not owned by the publisher.

Library of Congress Cataloging-in-Publication Data

Names: Jobson, Meghan, author. | Morgan, Juliet (Psychiatrist), author.
Title: Long illness: a practical guide to surviving, healing, and thriving / Meghan Jobson, MD, PhD, and Juliet Morgan, MD.
Description: First edition. | New York: Hachette Go, 2023. | Includes bibliographical references and index.
Identifiers: LCCN 2022050983 | ISBN 9780306828744 (hardcover) |
    ISBN 9780306828751 (paperback) | ISBN 9780306828768 (ebook)
Subjects: LCSH: Chronic diseases—Popular works. | Chronic diseases—Alternative treatment.
Classification: LCC RC108 .J63 2023 | DDC 616/.044—dc23/eng/20221214
LC record available at https://lccn.loc.gov/2022050983

ISBNs: 9780306828744 (hardcover); 9780306828768 (ebook)

Printed in the United States of America

LSC-C

Printing 1, 2023

Contents

PART IV
Long-Term Solutions and Lifestyle Medicine

Introduction
From Long Covid to
All Long Illness—You Are Not Alone

When the Covid-19 pandemic hit, stories about long Covid started coming out. News reports presented it like this was some new phenomenon: that not everyone is cured or recovers from illness. For those of us who have been sick, this story was nothing new. While some of the manifestations of long Covid may have some unique elements, the experience that people are having, of intense uncertainty, of renegotiating their identity, of rapidly having to discover both the successes and the massive failures of our health care system, those are not at all unique.

Long Covid has provided the health care system with a much-needed wake-up call: that we need a better way to deal with these sorts of illnesses, and the people who live with them need better support, better access to care, better education of our practitioners. We need the medical community to wake up and acknowledge that science doesn't know the answer to everything yet, and that's okay. We need more patient-led and patient-centered care. I am hopeful that things can change; I am hopeful that a twenty-year-old today might have a better relationship with illness than I did at that age because of the wisdom gained from others' experiences.

—JD, long illness survivor

*L*ong *illnesses are nothing new.* And they can happen to anyone. *What you are experiencing is real.* Millions of people like you live with illnesses that don't completely go away. Long illnesses are post-infectious, rheumatologic, autoimmune, neurologic, and inflammatory. Some have a clear diagnosis, and others do not. Many illnesses are "diagnoses of exclusion," meaning that they fall outside of conventional biomedical categories of understanding.

Although not all long illnesses are the same, many manifest themselves in similar ways. They can follow the same patterns in the body as a result of inflammation, trauma, nervous system imbalance, and toxic stress.

We treat and care for patients with long illnesses—illnesses like yours—every day. Using the science of conventional biomedicine supplemented with an expansive tool kit for healing, we watch our resilient clients reduce symptoms, find answers, learn new ways to cope, and reclaim their lives.

For years we have advocated for more attention to long illness and pushed back against a system not built to care for the clients we care for the most. Our specialty is long illness, which includes central sensitization syndromes, autoimmune disease, post-infectious syndromes, chronic inflammation, and pain (to name a few). *Long Covid brought other long illnesses out from the shadows.* After Covid-19 infections during the pandemic that began in 2020, people weren't getting better. They got worse, suffering headaches, fatigue, dizziness, shortness of breath, depression, and despair. Millions of previously healthy people were now sick, disabled, and alone. But for the first time in the history of long illnesses, other people started paying attention.

These illnesses require more than a conventional medical approach. Treating them requires addressing the roots of illness, not just the symptoms, and practitioners who view the body as interconnected in both visible and invisible ways.

Who Are We?

We are integrative physician-healers dedicated to working with people with long illness. Our work with long Covid opened the door to sharing our philosophies and practical approaches to recovery with all long illness sufferers.

We trained at top medical institutions, but building a skill set to treat our patients required seeking out experiences beyond the traditional medical tracks. Combined, we have completed three medical residencies, one PhD, three fellowships, and additional training in exercise physiology, mind-body medicine, psychedelic medicine, nutrition, and energy medicine. We have scoured the medical literature and philosophies from around the world. All of this work has been carried out in the pursuit of more answers, tools, and understanding for our patients, for our communities, and for ourselves. We journey alongside our patients. The recommendations in this book reflect what we practice in our clinics and in our own lives. We use integrative medicine in our own health care and in our families.

During the Covid-19 pandemic we developed an integrative medicine skills group for Covid recovery. It rapidly transformed into a group for treating long Covid. One thing became clear: there was significant overlap with the diseases we had treated in our clinics prior to the arrival of Covid-19. When working with this group, we used the skills and concepts for healing that we had put into practice across the full spectrum of disease. It quickly became clear that our group had to reach people suffering from more than long Covid. We needed to give people the experience of our philosophy of care so that they could apply it to *any* long illness. As in our clinics, the methods of care detailed in this book can be used by anyone struggling with a long illness.

An Integrative Approach

Our approach is anchored in evidence-based integrative medicine. Healing is not dependent on pharmaceuticals. Integrative medicine addresses the whole person: body, mind, and spirit.

In your experience, you might have felt like practitioners focus only on what's on the surface of your health. We explore what is underneath, helping you to strengthen your nervous system, reduce inflammation, and understand emotional connections.

This book will help you build a recovery tool kit. Recovery is a process, not always a destination. It is about reclaiming your identity, managing your symptoms, and becoming empowered to build the care team you deserve. We gather resources from biomedicine, psychotherapy, traditional Eastern medicines, nutrition, and mindfulness practices. You will also find expert opinions on topics like mitochondrial health, detoxification, brain

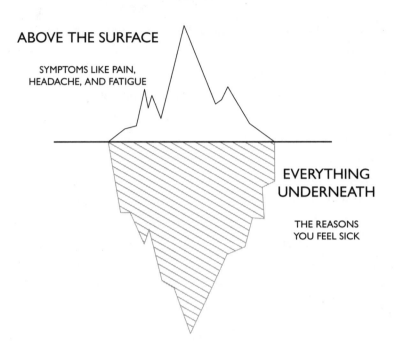

ABOVE THE SURFACE

SYMPTOMS LIKE PAIN,
HEADACHE, AND FATIGUE

EVERYTHING
UNDERNEATH

THE REASONS
YOU FEEL SICK

fog, and self-healing techniques. We acknowledge what is known and what is unknown. You will find no misinformation or "wallet toxicity" (expensive treatments that have little to no benefit) here. We use evidence to inform our recommendations and keep budgets and costs in mind.

We have also included exercises and journaling prompts. You may want to use a journal, notebook, or app to record your thoughts and respond to the exercises; you can keep a document on your computer or use your phone—whatever works best for you. We offer this book as a different kind of interactive experience. By the end of it, you will be equipped with data, self-knowledge, and integrative medicine skills. From our clinical experience, these are the ingredients needed to accelerate healing from within.

There's one more crucial ingredient: Healing happens when we feel less alone, so we have made sure to weave survivor stories throughout the book. You'll find their words anchoring chapters and supporting our suggestions. They are anonymous, but know that these survivors range in age, economic status, race, and sex. They have shared their stories in the hope that you will know you are not alone.

How to Use This Book

You can use this book in any way that feels right for you. If you read it consecutively, chapter by chapter, your knowledge and skills will layer. This is probably the most comprehensive way to build your personalized healing tool kit.

If reading the book this way doesn't feel right, skip to what you need. If you want help *now* with fatigue, skip to Chapter 5. If you are looking to make dietary changes tailored to your specific symptoms, open up to Chapter 18. Maybe you don't want to read medical and scientific explanations. That's okay. Jump to the journaling and skills sections within each chapter. You may need to process your experiences and gain skills first. If these are the sections that are calling to you, they are probably what you need the most. There is no right way to engage with these materials, only what is right for you. *There are no rules to this book, only resources.*

If you are sick and not getting better, you are in the right place. We have built a comprehensive resource for you. Join us as we build your tool kit for recovery together.

PART I

FOUNDATIONS

You may already have a diagnosis or diagnoses; you may have been feeling unwell for a long time or your symptoms are new. Regardless of where you are, this part will help you to understand a bit about all long illnesses, as well as look at the big picture of long illness (in short: it affects many of us—and as we'll repeat throughout, you are not alone), healthcare, and disability. It will also empower you to choose the best healthcare partners for you.

CHAPTER I

What Long Illness Is, What Causes It, and What It Can Mean for You

In March of 2020, my wife and I both had Covid.

Then, about three months later, I began to have these new experiences: increase in fatigue, shortness of breath, headaches, and memory loss. My emotional state was being impacted by all this; I felt very alone.

Joining a support group had a very deep positive effect on my recovery. Now, two or three times a week, I'll sit out on the deck. I do meditation practices; I review the exercises. I look at how I cope with the stress and the physical challenges that I've been dealing with. And I just try to remind myself of the tools and skills I learned. Having them all [mindfulness, journaling, coping skills] is important. And each of them contributes individually, but doing these activities collectively is what makes a big difference. I say recovery—I'm not recovered yet, but I'm showing signs. I realized that I'm not alone in this. That there are support systems out there. And I think that it's really the combined efforts.

Before we get to any nuts and bolts, we want to share with you something that guides every page of this book: long illness includes anyone who identifies with the symptoms described here. You don't have to have a certain diagnosis to qualify. *This book is for anyone who is suffering and looking for a whole-body, psychologically informed understanding and treatment of illness.*

What You Will Learn in This Chapter:

- The definition of long illness
- Common causes of long illness

- A comprehensive overview of inflammation and its relationship to long illness
- An overview and explanation of the tools and methods you will explore in this book

What Is a Long Illness?

The term *long illness* represents a paradigm shift. There are hundreds of long illnesses, all with different names, but they can show up in the body in similar ways and be caused by the same underlying problems. Let's review a list of common diagnoses that fall under the umbrella of a long illness before exploring what this means and how it applies to you:

Addison's disease	Dysautonomia	Migraines
Alzheimer's disease	Ehlers-Danlos syndrome	Multiple sclerosis
Ankylosing spondylitis	Encephalitis	Myalgic encephalomyelitis (CFS)
Arthritis	Endometriosis	Nervous system disorders
Asthma	Epilepsy	Obsessive-compulsive disorder
Bipolar disorder	Fibromyalgia	Post-traumatic stress disorder
Brain injury/concussions	Generalized anxiety	Psoriasis
Cancer	Genetic syndromes	Rheumatoid arthritis
Celiac disease	Heart disease	Schizophrenia
Chronic and post-Lyme	Heart failure	Scleroderma
Chronic kidney disease	Hepatitis	Shingles
Chronic lung disease	HIV/AIDS	Stroke
Cystic fibrosis	Immune system disorders	Systemic lupus erythematosus
Dementia	Inflammatory bowel disease	Thyroiditis
Depression	Irritable bowel disease	Trauma
Diabetes	Long Covid	Tremor

You may identify with more than one diagnosis. Many of them overlap and are connected because of underlying inflammation, autoimmunity, or nervous system dysfunction. Or you may be sick without a diagnosis. You too will find answers here.

"Long illness" is a term we use for illnesses that don't improve on a short time line. An illness may linger for several months, then resolve. It might get better, then worse. It might recur in cycles, or it could last for years. Some symptoms might worsen, while others improve. It could flare with stress or emotional upheaval. All of these patterns are seen across the wide spectrum of long illness.

You may have one diagnosis that supposedly identified a single problem, but it doesn't fully explain the way you are feeling. For example, you may have been diagnosed with depression, but it's your body, not your mind, that feels like it's falling apart. This makes sense to us. Depression can increase the sympathetic nervous system's fight-or-flight response, which leads the body to be on guard and causes imbalances in multiple organ systems. Depression also increases inflammation and can have symptoms that emerge throughout the body, including bloating, constipation, memory problems, brain fog, headaches, and fatigue (among others). Or your depression may be secondary to another process that has gone undiagnosed. Long illness requires an acknowledgment of the intimate relationship between mind and body and the need for bringing the full force of integrative medicine to treatment. This is a different kind of care than what is typically offered for depression alone.

Another example is arthritis. Arthritis of any kind results from and causes increased inflammation, which has consequences throughout the body. Arthritis pain can worsen your mood and reduce your ability to move your body, which can increase inflammation and cause imbalances in the nervous system. Again, you may have been diagnosed with one problem, arthritis, but it can have any number of symptoms throughout your body. A diagnosis of arthritis alone doesn't explain why you feel fatigued, have bloating and diarrhea, and can't get to sleep. A single label doesn't do justice to your experience. You have a long illness.

We believe that very few illnesses are "isolated," existing on their own without impacting the whole body. Our health care system is misguided in treating illness as a single entity and taking medication-only approaches. Long illnesses respond best to treatments that consider the whole body and underlying causes.

Why did we choose to call them "long illnesses" and not "chronic illnesses"? The trend of changing the way we look at and define illness began with long Covid, which was named by people who had the disease, not by medical professionals looking for a quick label. "Chronic," for us, feels stagnant. It also carries an intense stigma from a medical establishment that prizes procedures over personalized care. "Long" acknowledges uncertainty and avoids dismissive terms like "post" and "syndrome," which can delegitimize suffering. As we said earlier, "long illness" includes anyone who identifies with it. We honor and validate your experience.

One of the first steps is to get a better understanding of the causes or roots of your illness, whether it's one primary cause with others layered on top or a cluster of causes. It can be useful to reflect on what you suspect or believe are the roots of your illness. Throughout this book we will be explaining these roots further and referring to them. Here we will provide simply a very general overview.

Common Causes of Long Illness

Allergy: Some people are allergic to things in their environment, or to foods. By reducing exposure, their symptoms improve. But for others the allergy system in the body can become overactive and produce allergic responses even in the absence of exposure to a clear allergen.

Autoimmunity: The body can begin to not recognize parts of itself and to treat them as if they are foreign. Autoimmune illnesses can target one organ in the body (isolated) or be widespread (systemic). Autoimmunity can arise spontaneously or after an infection or other illness.

Central sensitization: The nervous system begins to interpret signals from the environment as amplified, resulting in pain from input that wouldn't normally be painful.

Endocrine: Hormone balance is essential for body regulation (*homeostasis*). When hormones become unbalanced, the effects are systemic. Common hormone imbalances include elevated thyroid levels, decreased sex hormone levels, and stress hormone shifts.

Environmental: Past or current exposure to environmental toxins can overload pathways in the body and set off a cascade of problems.

Genetic: Genes carry vulnerabilities and predispositions to long illness. This is especially apparent in families with many members who have a long illness. Genes can also change over time and be impacted by the environment in what is called epigenetic change.

Infectious/post-infectious: Long illnesses caused by infections can occur through a number of mechanisms, including ongoing infection, reactivation of the infection, post-infectious damage, and secondary autoimmune reactions triggered by infection. Some infections can be suppressed or cleared by targeted therapies, but many others cannot. Many mystery illnesses are triggered by infection. For example, recent evidence suggests that mononucleosis (EBV infection) may be the leading cause of multiple sclerosis, and it has been implicated in the development of long Covid. With research dollars now being poured into long Covid, we are learning more about all of these post-infectious syndromes every day.

Inflammation: Increased inflammation in the body can come from many different sources and may or may not show up on laboratory studies. Inflammation is the body's healing mechanism, which can go awry. Inflammation plays a part in most long illnesses. It is a cause rather than a symptom.

Malignancy: Cancer, either occurring presently or in your history, can have ripple effects throughout the body. The same is true of cancer treatments, which are often life-saving but take a tremendous toll on the body.

Metabolic/mitochondrial: Metabolism and energy production by mitochondria are implicated in many long illnesses.

Nervous system dysfunction: Your nervous system runs from your brain to your fingertips and toes. Disruption in your nervous system can affect any part of your body, from memory and mood to heart rate, digestion, balance, and pain. For most people with long illness there is a neurologic element, while others identify a neurologic illness as the root (*primary diagnosis*) of their long illness.

Post-traumatic response: An accident or an injury in the body triggers a cascade of symptoms that can have an impact long after the initial event. The same is true for psychological trauma.

Psychological: Emotional health is health. Challenges to mental health can increase inflammation and change pathways in the brain that contribute to symptoms throughout the body.

Vascular: Blockages, clots, and inflammation of blood vessels can contribute to or cause long illness.

This is by no means an exhaustive list, but it includes the most common roots of long illness that come up repeatedly in our patients' experience. Sometimes one clear trigger sets off a cascade of symptoms. Here is a common example:

Infection → post-infectious syndrome → autoimmunity → inflammation → central sensitization

This person experiences fatigue, body aches, painful joints, irritable bowel syndrome, and dysautonomia. Here is another example:

Concussion → nervous system dysfunction → central sensitization → inflammation → post-traumatic pain (migraines)

This person experiences fatigue, dysautonomia, depression, and migraines.

The most common pattern for most people with long illness is a feeling that all of the causes are linked and lumped together, so their recovery plan has to address multiple causes and roots.

Inflammation

Inflammation can be a good thing. It is how our bodies heal when we get injured or develop an infection. Humans' strong inflammatory response allowed our ancestors to survive. But in modern times we can have *too much* of a good thing. When the inflammatory system responds too much or for too long, the result is chronic, systemic inflammation. When this happens, instead of helping, inflammation makes us unwell.

Chronic inflammation is like an out-of-control party inside your body. Remember that little party you threw (or thought about throwing) while your parents were away in high school? Although it began with good intentions, after your friends invited their friends and their friends invited their own friends, too many people showed up and the party ended in a big mess (see any teen movie for a refresher). That's what chronic inflammation does inside your body.

When you get an infection or injury, a signal is released that tells the immune cells hanging out nearby that there is an injury. Once the inflammation signal is sent, your body, focused on survival and recovery, first sends energy and nutrients to the injured area. During this time, you experience symptoms that we call *sickness behaviors*, like resting more, eating less, and spending less time with others. These symptoms show that your body is conserving energy for healing, and it's a common experience for anyone who ever got the flu or broke a bone. Our bodies have evolved these behaviors so that we will survive. If that signal doesn't go away, however, your body will continue to focus energy on the areas of inflammation. If you have a whole-body illness, this could mean that inflammation is happening everywhere. Over time the continued whole-body inflammation can result in muscle loss, thinning bones, anemia, metabolism changes, high blood pressure, changes in blood sugar, and more.

For many who have long illnesses, these symptoms could be signs of a flare of their disease. The good news is that almost no matter what is triggering the underlying inflammation, and no matter how severe it is, there are tools that can help.

Flares

Whether you are flaring or in a state of well-controlled disease, it is important that you take an inflammation inventory periodically to make sure that you are doing what you can to maintain your well-being. Always check with your practitioners to determine whether you are having a flare of your existing conditions or need screening to rule out an alternative treatable diagnosis. You didn't choose to have a long illness, but you can make choices to decrease your inflammation.

What Causes Chronic Inflammation?

We have little control over some things, like our genetics, exposures to toxins, and illnesses. Moreover, chronic inflammation often has more than one cause or there is more than one contribution to it. Are any of these common conditions familiar to your experience?

Persistent infection	Caused either by difficult-to-eradicate organisms or organisms that are resistant to the treatment you were given, for example, fungus, bacteria, or viruses
Autoimmune disease	Your immune system sees a part of your body as foreign and attacks it, for example, in psoriasis or rheumatoid arthritis
Recurrent episodes of acute inflammation	Caused by repeated or recurrent infections, injury, abuse, or stressful life events (see Chapter 16)
Irritant or foreign material exposure	Usually coming from the environment, especially work exposures such as coal, asbestos, or silica
Auto-inflammatory disease	Inflammation cells can't turn off appropriately, as in familial Mediterranean fever or hyper IgE syndrome; rare, usually inherited, and starts in childhood, but can also be acquired later in life
Mitochondrial dysfunction	The part of the cell that provides energy can't work well, causing the cell to send signals that increase inflammation (see Chapter 17)

Inflammation increases as we age because of natural changes in how our cells manage energy. Fat cells release chemical signals called *cytokines*, which can worsen inflammation. For those with long illness, disease flares and the persistent stress that surrounds illness can increase overall inflammation. The table illustrates some of the different factors that can affect levels of inflammation in your body.

Increases Inflammation	Decreases Inflammation
Poor sleep	Practice meditation, yoga, or breathing
High work stress	Higher level of physical activity
Poverty	Lower body fat
Lower subjective social status	Greater kindness to self
Increased loneliness	Healthy reflective thinking
Increased social isolation	Ability to see both sides
Anger	Minimal to no substance use
Low self-esteem	Nonsmoker or former smoker
Poor quality of life	Plant-based diet
Difficult or traumatic childhood	A childhood spent with animals in a rural environment

Lists like this can feel overwhelming. The point here is to shine a light on the often unspoken burdens that many of us carry. Some of them can't be changed. Our message is not that you must address every aspect of your life perfectly; it's that you can make small changes to your daily habits, thoughts, and routines that can have profound effects on the level of inflammation in your body.

How Do You Know If You Have Chronic Inflammation?

Chronic inflammation is common, but the underlying cause can be different in every person who experiences it. It accompanies many conditions ranging from autoimmune disease to heart and lung disease. If you have been diagnosed with a chronic condition, there is some degree of chronic inflammation in your body already. Even with well-controlled disease or without a diagnosis, there are some common symptoms that people with chronic inflammation experience:

Fatigue	Low energy	Depression	Anxiety
Mood issues	Bad PMS, periods	Constipation	Diarrhea
Acid reflux	Bloating	Abdominal pain	Balance issues
Weight gain	Weight loss	Recurrent infections	Low back pain

Rashes	Swollen lymph nodes	Difficulty sleeping	Body pain
Muscle pain	Joint pain	Brain fog	Difficulty concentrating
Blurred vision	Dry eyes and mouth	Memory issues	Headaches
High blood pressure	Water retention	Fevers or chills	Cough and sore throat
Runny or stuffy nose	Hives	Shortness of breath	Low sex drive

Once chronic inflammation is identified, we focus on integrative treatment, including powerful tools and lifestyle modifications to decrease inflammation.

External Influences on Health

Your health is more than a lab value or a symptom. It is a complex mix of genetics, environment, and personal history. Racist and sexist systems and other factors like education level, poverty, and community characteristics all contribute to the state of your health. Some people argue that your zip code makes as big a contribution to your health as your genetic code. All of these contributions to your health are called *social determinants of health.*

We wish that all of our readers with a long illness had the same experience navigating it, but they don't. Any difference in your experience can reduce the chance that you will receive the care you need to heal.

For our readers of color, we recognize that you face additional barriers. Not all books about health are written for you or reflect your experiences. Dr. Rita Crooms, a neurologist and lecturer on racial disparities in medicine at Mount Sinai Medical Center, explains:

> We need to emphasize the impact of racism and social inequity on long illness and overall health. Racism may affect many aspects of health, from social and environmental factors that increase the risk of disease to the care that is provided once someone becomes ill. These and other systemic inequities disproportionately affecting communities of color can put them at higher risk for health problems long before they become ill and make it more difficult to return to a state of health.

For people who become ill, racial disparities can affect not only access to health care, but also the type of care they receive, how their illness is managed, and their likelihood of being included in research that will help others with the disease.

Long illness doesn't discriminate, but this book seeks to empower readers of all racial and ethnic backgrounds to take charge of their health through greater understanding of long illness.

Gender bias also has an impact on people's experiences with long illness. Women are disproportionately affected by long illnesses such as long Covid, chronic fatigue syndrome, and fibromyalgia. In fact, autoimmunity in general is more common in women. There are also differences for some people of color, who experience higher rates of several long illnesses linked to autoimmunity, most notably systemic lupus erythematosus (SLE), myalgic encephalomyelitis/chronic fatigue syndrome (ME/CFS), and rheumatoid arthritis. There are also risks for LGBTQIA+ individuals, including elevated rates of some cancers and depression.

This book includes diverse survivor stories from people of different racial, gender, and economic backgrounds. The physicians quoted in this book also reflect the diversity we believe is critical to bringing about the changes that need to happen in medicine.

Uncertainty and Invalidation

There's just so many unknowns. And you're trying to get a handle on what therapies will actually work for it. That's trial and error. How long is it gonna take to get well?

Long illnesses linger. They can persist for months, improve and worsen in cycles, or last a lifetime. And often one of the hardest parts of a long illness is the uncertainty. You may be suffering, but have few answers. You may feel a little better, but then you feel worse. Nobody will tell you how long the illness will last. For many, there are no medications specifically designed for their disease. Or the medications and treatments on offer thus far have brought incomplete relief.

In this book, we will work with you to navigate this uncertainty and keep moving toward healing. It will be important as we do so to balance the things we don't know with the things we *do* know.

> *There's a lot of talk about "it's in your head." I had a lot of tests done where everything came back normal. My ANA [antinuclear antibodies test] came back normal. I don't have these markers in my blood work for inflammation. I had doctors tell me, "You shouldn't be feeling so bad, because there's nothing going on." It's not just in my head, and it does make you question like: Is it real? Is it in my head? I really don't think it is.*

Another difficulty with long illness is that people are often told, when their symptoms cannot yet be explained, that what they are experiencing isn't real. You may have been told this in ways that are clear—as when a practitioner brushes off your questions—or ways that are more subtle, as when a family member questions your fatigue *again*.

These messages are invalidating and demoralizing. Over time you may have stopped trusting yourself. That only makes it harder to hear what your body needs to heal.

We trust that you are the expert on your own body. In this book, we are partnering with you on your path to healing. Listen to what your body needs from this book and move toward it. Use this book in any way that feels right for you.

Defining Medicine

Throughout the book, we'll refer to different types of medicine:

Conventional medicine: Also called allopathic, Western, mainstream, orthodox, or biomedicine, conventional medicine is a system that uses doctors, nurses, and other health care professionals to diagnose and treat disease with pharmaceuticals, surgery, and various therapies.

Traditional medicine: Also called complementary, alternative, or holistic medicine, traditional medicine refers to practices that have been used for centuries, such as East Asian medicine. Some traditional practices have been so thoroughly tested that they are now considered mainstream conventional medicine. Chapter 20 is devoted to traditional medicine and how it can support you on your long illness journey.

Integrative medicine: The practice of using the biomedical model of evidence-based medicine, with special training in traditional practices. As we mentioned in the introduction, this is the type of medicine we practice and the type that informs this book. Considering the increasing prevalence of people who use what is sometimes referred to as complementary or alternative medicine (CAM), it is important to have physicians who are trained and knowledgeable in these systems. Physicians who fully understand how and when to use CAM in a beneficial way are better able to teach their patients the most healthful way to use this approach.

Why Use Integrative Medicine in Long Illness?

As physicians, we are trained in conventional biomedicine. We use in-depth knowledge of anatomy and physiology to diagnose our patients' problems. Our primary tool for treatment is medication. This type of medicine works well in many settings, especially places like an intensive care unit or emergency room. *But on its own, conventional biomedicine falls short in treating chronic illness.*

Integrative medicine centers on the patient. It is open-minded and holistic. While we practice conventional biomedicine, we also use natural products, traditional healing philosophies, and mind-body medicine. This expanded skill set has helped us provide better care for our patients with complex diseases.

We encourage you to explore and learn a variety of techniques. All of our recommendations come from medical evidence and are cost-conscious. You can implement many of the treatments, like mindfulness exercises, at home. We also have a guide to building your own medical team, which is especially helpful if you live far away from a specialty center.

We believe in combining the best parts of biomedicine with traditional medicines. This book integrates both worlds to maximize your knowledge and expand your tool kit for healing.

Foundational Tools

Mindfulness

Mindfulness is a practice of "tuning in" and becoming aware of your body. It is also an opportunity to tune out the rest of the world. You may think that mindfulness is complicated or only for people who have time to do little else. But mindfulness is something you do for *you*. It can be a moment of breath in your home.

We are confident about recommending mindfulness because of the evidence we have about its impact on multiple long illnesses. Mindfulness has been shown to reduce symptoms of depression, improve energy levels in patients with chronic fatigue, and reduce pain for those suffering from fibromyalgia.

We are also confident about its efficacy because so many of our patients and support group members have told us that mindfulness works for them. Most say that mindfulness reduces stress and anxiety. It gives them a few minutes of quiet and a chance to recharge their system. For many, it also reduces headaches, improves fatigue, and makes breathing more comfortable.

In this book, we will offer you different ways to be mindful. Our exercises are approximately five minutes long. They do not require props or they cost nothing. Mindfulness has no risks or side effects, but it does have powerful effects on the mind and body. For the best results, we recommend that you practice mindfulness daily.

Mindfulness has been used by those with lung conditions like asthma and chronic obstructive pulmonary disease. Some people with shortness of breath, however, hesitate to do exercises that focus on breathing. If you are one of them, listen to your body. If your body says no, listen to it. If you are hesitant about mindfulness but open to it, try making modifications, like lying down or shortening the exercise. It can be hard to be mindful when something about the practice feels difficult, so be gentle on yourself. Try these skills at the edge of your comfort zone, but listen to your body.

If you like the mindfulness exercises in this book, we strongly recommend exploring other resources and deepening your practice. One program we highly recommend is called *mindfulness-based stress reduction* (MBSR). This is an eight-week program run through some community organizations and universities. We also like several meditation apps. If five minutes feels good, why not try practicing for a longer period? We have information on how to expand your exposure to mindfulness in the resources section at the back of the book.

How Does Mindfulness Work?

When you feel a threat, it revs up the fight-or-flight engine of your nervous system, also known as the *sympathetic nervous system.*

When the sympathetic nervous system is turned on, almost every organ in your body is affected: your heart rate increases, your lungs expand, your eyes dilate, and your stomach rumbles. Your body also pumps out a stress hormone called *cortisol.* This system evolved to allow us to escape predators, but it isn't built for long-term stress.

When stress lasts for months or even years, this system meant to protect you starts to work against your body. When stress hormones remain high, you feel exhausted. Being in a constant state of fight-or-flight causes prolonged stress on your body and prevents you from fully relaxing. Almost every organ in your body is affected. Such chronic stress can weaken your immune system and impair your memory.

Mindfulness strengthens the other half of your nervous system, the "rest-and-digest" *parasympathetic nervous system.* This system counteracts the fight-or-flight response and brings the body into balance. We spend most of our lives listening to the world outside of our bodies. Mindfulness has us tune *in* instead. It may feel uncomfortable to slow down. It may feel boring. It may make you aware of how much stress your body is holding. These are normal reactions. As we guide you in exploring mindfulness, remember that you can practice for just a few moments a day. Just keep practicing. It will get better.

EXERCISE

MINDFULNESS

Your inner voice, or what some call *intuition*, is a guide to healing. Following this inner voice will help you maximize the healing potential of this book. This exercise is designed to strengthen that connection.

We will do this by repeating a simple phrase, what some refer to as chanting a *mantra*. Mantras have been used in scientific studies to improve well-being and have been shown to produce more relaxed brain waves. We will be using mantras as a way to communicate with your intuition. We chant to tell the body, "I am listening to you. I am caring for you. I am healing you."

Read through the mantras below. See if there is one that makes you feel more connected to yourself and your healing journey. This choice may be clear, or it may not. That's okay. You can practice with any of the phrases or make one up for yourself. Here are a few examples:

"I trust"

"I listen"

"I heal"

Once you have chosen a mantra, set a timer for five minutes. Breathe slowly. Every two to three breaths, repeat your phrase, either inside your head or out loud.

When you are done, open your eyes. Know that you have taken another step toward understanding what your body needs. We will continue to strengthen this connection as we move along in this book.

Journaling

Writing in a journal is a way to get to know your own mind. Expressing your thoughts and feelings in writing has been shown to reduce anxiety and distress. You will see journaling exercises throughout this book. You can use the journaling prompt or just write whatever is on your mind. Your thoughts and feelings are important. Those exercises invite you to process anything that comes up for you. Let's start with these prompts:

What do I need from this book?

How do I plan to use this book?

Psychological Skills and Exercises

Long illness is a complex tapestry; your recovery will be incomplete if you do not pay enough attention to the connection between your emotional life and your physical body. The brain is like a superhighway system. The neural networks that control emotions, pain, and movement are like roads. We think of these networks as separate roads, but they are actually connected. When one of these "roads" is busy and traffic backs up, a car may take an exit it never meant to take. This is how stress turns into headaches, pain, or worsening fatigue.

Not all pain and fatigue stem from an overloaded emotional pathway. Far from it. Emotional overload can contribute to preexisting symptoms in the body. Stress and anxiety can make a headache worse. Suppressed anger and resentment are exhausting. And long illness causes even the most balanced individuals to experience insecurity, anxiety, and feelings of being overwhelmed.

Changing the brain changes the body. Developing your psychological skills can help you offload your emotional pathways, support your ways of coping, and increase your understanding of the connections between your body and mind. We address psychological skills in several ways. One of them is by incorporating exercises from several major schools of therapy, many of them inspired by a form of therapy called *cognitive behavioral therapy* (CBT).

CBT stresses the connections between your thoughts, feelings, and behaviors, usually by helping you change your thinking patterns, understand how you cope, and set goals for recovery. CBT is the most common type of therapy exercise in this book because we have substantial evidence for its use in treating numerous illnesses, from chronic fatigue syndrome to depression and migraine.

EXERCISE

COGNITIVE BEHAVIORAL THERAPY

Listening deeply to your inner voice can help you heal. Unfortunately, that's harder than ever to do when you feel sick and find it hard to feel like yourself anymore. You have many strengths, however, and others probably see them readily.

This exercise will help you remember who you are on the inside, reminding you that you have many strengths, even though you are sick. Tapping into your strengths can help you feel stronger and more willing to try new things.

Look at the strengths listed here. Which ones stand out for you? They may be strengths you see in yourself or strengths that other people see in you. If you are having trouble, ask a family member or friend to help. What other strengths do you have that are not listed here? Write them down, and when you are done, look at your list and take a moment to honor these strengths inside of yourself.

Trustworthy	Adventurous	Optimistic	Wise
Creative	Artistic	Funny	Compassionate
Flexible	Kind	Open-minded	Smart
Curious	Laid back	Thoughtful	Intuitive

CHAPTER 2

Your Life with Long Illness

At first, the experience of illness can make you feel like you've become the disease. When you first understand that long illness is setting in, you may worry that you'll never be yourself again. Many struggle with this new existence because initially, compared to life before long illness, it just feels like a struggle. No one wants to be sick, and especially not like this.

With support, self-compassion, and time, you can navigate toward understanding yourself in a new and different way—not necessarily as better or worse, but as different. Some people might see the illness as the most important part of their identity, while for others it's just one of many aspects of who they are. Disruptions to your identity can alter your self-image, your self-esteem, and your sense of how you fit into the world around you. Illness can make you feel isolated and overwhelmed. For most humans, any kind of change is hard. It's important to remember that you are not alone, and that there are others having similar experiences.

What You Will Learn in This Chapter:

- The different impacts of illness on identity
- An understanding of how the world around you relates to illness and how it may be affecting you
- That disability applies broadly to anyone with an illness who identifies with the long illness experience, and that there are accommodations for disability
- How to build a health care team around you

Illness identity refers to the degree to which a chronic health condition becomes a person's identity. There are four main paths that person might take during the course of their illness: engulfment, rejection, acceptance, and enrichment. Read over the descriptions of these four paths. You might notice that you have taken more than one of these paths during your illness, or that different paths have merged to create your experience. Before responding to "Things to Think About," first ask yourself how you are feeling today. Then think back: How is the way you feel today different from how you felt when you first were sick and at different points in your illness experience? Looking forward, can you imagine how your illness identity may or may not change?

Dimensions of Illness Identity	What It Means	Things to Think About

Engulfment: Being "swallowed up" by your illness	People who are engulfed in their illness feel that their illness has taken over their identity. They visit practitioners more often, experience depression, anxiety, and physical symptoms at higher levels, and are more likely to be hospitalized than similar people with the same illness. These people are more likely to report a lower quality of life and a higher degree of distress, as well as to have severe symptoms and side effects.
	    Higher emotional distress
	    More drug side effects and more severe symptoms
	    Lower health-related quality of life
		How much does your long illness dominate your identity and daily life?

Rejection	Higher levels of rejection make people less likely to optimally self-manage their illness. The most extreme cases deny that they have any health issues. Since they are unlikely to treat their illness, they tend to report more severe physical symptoms. They are also more likely to miss school or work.
	    Lower life satisfaction
	    Higher emotional distress
	    Greater chance of other identity issues (such as around relationship building or education)
		Do you reject your long illness as part of your identity? If so, how much? Why?

Acceptance	People who are able to accept that their health has changed have less severe symptoms and side effects and are less upset by their health changes. They tend to have fewer mental and physical symptoms of disease and are more likely to adhere to their treatment plan. 　　Fewer drug side effects and lessened 　　　severity of symptoms 　　Lower emotional distress 　　Higher life satisfaction	Do you accept your long illness as part of your identity? How much?
Enrichment	Those in the adaptive state of enrichment are more likely to have improved adaptive psychological functioning. Because they are more likely to adhere to treatment over time, they are less likely to feel they are in a state of engulfment. The positive stress-related changes they make are more strongly correlated with positive psychological outcomes. 　　Increased life satisfaction 　　Lower emotional distress 　　More likely to visit their primary care 　　　practitioner	Does your long illness enrich your life? Have you made positive lifestyle changes? Has your outlook on life changed for the better? How?

Your perception of your illness has a greater impact on your condition than other factors such as depression, physical functioning, and pain levels. Working with practitioners, loved ones, and your illness community to modify your perceptions about your illness can significantly improve your well-being.

Journaling

SELF-IDENTITY

Who are you? What are the different roles that you play in your life? Listed here are some types of responsibility you might have in your day-to-day life. Write out this list in your journal and then think about your activities yesterday, last month, last year. What type of responsibility characterizes these activities?

Your activities and responsibilities make up your self-identity, or how you see yourself in the world. Having a long illness can sometimes steal time away from these important aspects of your life.

Cultural	Health	Sexual
Disability	Interests and hobbies	Other
Ethnic, national	Occupational	
Gender	Religious	

Take a moment to think about what you spend your days doing and then journal your thoughts. What identities are easy for you to claim? Which ones are harder? How can you spend more time doing enriching activities that highlight the positive aspects of your self-identity?

I think about what it would mean if I wasn't sick. I think about how much time I would have left if I didn't have to sleep nine hours a night, if I didn't have to go to physical therapy, or go to the doctors' appointments. I think about all the emotional energy I expend thinking about how I feel about the fact that I am in pain, what information should I tell my supervisors at work, what do I need to cover up and when. What shoes can I wear for how long so I can walk? What pants won't bother my scars? All of the mental math I have to do every hour, it just seems unfair and more complicated than what other people my age are thinking about.

But then I think about what it has given me. I have been able to do research in disability and pain. I volunteer to be a peer mentor for others with my condition, which brings me so much fulfillment. Letting others know they are not alone is big for me, because I didn't know anyone else like me. My life has been enriched by these experiences. It has made me more patient with myself and others who are going through hard things.

How the World Sees Sick People

Let's say that you have it all together: you are accepting your illness and it is enriching your life. Now turn on the TV, pick up a book, watch a play, or listen to a song. How illness and disability are portrayed in our culture has come a long way in the last century, but we still have a long way to go. Many of these portrayals are still romanticized versions of what disability and illness look like, and at the end of the story the disabled person often either overcomes an obstacle to fit in with the "normal" crowd or dies. Many plots focus on their differences as a plot twist or as a terrible burden to overcome, and disabled people are rarely featured in rom-coms or scary movies. In literature and films, the sick and disabled are represented largely by outdated tropes. Most annoying for those with long illness is the myth of the ill or disabled person who is miraculously cured or whose mere existence is a moving inspiration to those who cannot imagine living the life of the unwell. Newer media are working on changing these depictions, but it can be overwhelming to see the contrast between your life and the stereotypes of your illness.

During much of the Covid-19 pandemic, the public messages were stressful for people with chronic illnesses, who were told that their illness might make them more likely to get Covid-19 or to have severe complications, including death. Despite the fact that a large portion of the world's population has a chronic illness or disability, the message from news outlets and officials was that it was safe for people to go without masks unless they were sick. The dismissal of the chronically ill as disposable is all too common, and the pandemic just highlighted some of the ways in which public health messaging could be made more inclusive. Such messaging is often aimed at people who are "healthy" and "able-bodied" and ignores the impact on the growing number of "others."

As the pandemic's impact shifted, a new group of chronically ill post-Covid and long Covid patients flooded health care systems, which were already unable to provide adequate care for many people with long or chronic illnesses. The volume and medical needs of those affected by Covid-19 down the road are likely to change how we approach long illnesses.

After my diagnosis I was like, maybe I'll be one of those people who runs a half-marathon on the one-year anniversary. It's because those are the narratives that we are given in our society; that the appropriate way to have a

different body is to overcome it, to conquer it. Therapy helped me realize, "Oh,
no, I don't get to overcome this. This is me now, and I have to make sense of
it." I gained strength from reading books about people with stories similar to
mine. Seeing how they claim their identities and journeys. I met others whose
identities were changing from illness and created a support network that way.
Learning more about illness and disability studies, reading books and learning
about the research, was empowering to me.

Diagnosis

When I got my first diagnosis, I was quite sure it was wrong. But I went from
being ignored and treated like I was crazy to my symptoms being taken seri-
ously and treatments being offered. I was so happy I was seen, I didn't care
what they did to me. They were wrong, and I was given harmful, pointless
treatments for years until I finally pushed to see a different type of doctor.
In the end, the most helpful treatments for my disease are having supportive
doctors and therapists and mostly trying to have the healthiest lifestyle I can
maintain. Sleep, good diet, happy relationships, a nice walk in the sunshine,
and a good therapist have all helped me live a life that reduces my symptoms
enough where often I don't need loads of medication and therapies. This works
for every condition, so I am perplexed why they aren't given to everyone who
is struggling with difficult symptoms. Like, why do we spend so much time on
naming the disease and no time teaching us how to live a life that reduces the
pain our disease brings?

Our whole lives we hear the same beautiful story again and again: a vibrant
person experiences changes in their body that limit them, no one knows
how to help, a hero figure steps in and solves the problem, and then they
live happily ever after. We want to believe these stories because they offer
us hope if we, or people we love, are suffering from long illness. But these
myths can be harmful when they teach us that differences in our bodies are
problems that need to be fixed or solved.

Our current biomedical system of care has developed around these myths.
The media's limited views of illness are reinforced by how practitioners are

taught. To be fair, medical students must learn hundreds of years of data in a short time, and using stereotypes and well-known stories is one important way in which people learn. However, putting a person in a box with a diagnosis doesn't work all the time. Many long illnesses don't fit into these boxes. When your practitioner can't fit your symptoms into a diagnosis, you might feel dismissed or misunderstood. On behalf of your practitioner, we apologize. It is not their intention to make you feel that way. That this happens as often as it does is one of the many unfortunate side effects of the way much of modern health care is delivered, but that is beyond the scope of this book.

During your search for the right diagnosis, you might be sent to other medical centers with more expertise in your symptoms or more appropriate testing facilities. Even in these specialized practices you may experience negative interactions with practitioners. You should always seek out second and maybe third opinions. Medicine is a team sport. If only one practitioner thinks you have a particular condition and wants to treat you in a certain way, that should give you pause.

Some people who get the "right diagnosis" might feel happy after experiencing the sometimes isolating symptoms of long illness. Humans like naming things; the name of our illness helps us explain to other people what we are going through. A diagnosis validates our concerns and makes us feel like we were complaining for good reason. But a diagnosis isn't always all it's cracked up to be.

A diagnosis isn't a cure. Even with a diagnosis, illnesses rarely change overnight. You can have a constellation of symptoms that right now we call disease X and treat with treatments A, B, or C. But symptoms and diagnoses can change over time. Your symptoms are just as valid and real as they were before you had a label for them. And for some of you, treatment A, B, or C may not do as much to improve your quality of life as you had hoped.

On the other hand, having a diagnosis is very handy. You can get access and coverage for certain treatments in different health care systems. Maybe you can get a disabled person's license plate and a care aide or other assistance to help with tasks; maybe a diagnosis makes it easier to get a wheelchair paid for. These things add up. But having a diagnosis doesn't guarantee that your condition will get better, or that you will receive more respect now that your symptoms have a name.

> *Without a diagnosis, I am powerless. I'd rather have the wrong diagnosis and be seen, than be ignored and treated like I am crazy or annoying.*

> *I encourage people who are sick to think about a diagnosis as a tool. It is not a life sentence. Getting a diagnosis is the way to get resourced, and that's a good thing. And I would have wanted my younger self to know other people who are going through complex medical issues, and to find someone I can talk to about my illness, not necessarily the same illness, but someone I can share a similar language with. That has been really helpful and has left me feeling less alone. It helped me realize you can be two things at once. You can wish you didn't have to deal with the inconveniences of having a different body, while also accepting it as being an important part of who you are.*

"The question is not how to get cured, but how to live."[1] Post-diagnosis, you are the same person with the same symptoms. Hopefully, the treatments and support from your community will improve your quality of life. But there is a reason that we focus so much of this book on how to improve your daily choices and habits and how to manage complex symptoms. These changes will get you back on track and help you no matter what symptoms you have. Whether or not you have a diagnosis, and whether or not you're in treatment, you can improve your quality of life and your feeling of control and understanding of what is going on in your body.

Journaling

DIAGNOSIS

Have you been diagnosed?

How did the diagnosis make you feel? Did it change how you saw yourself?

What could have been different about how you were diagnosed that would have made it better or easier for you?

Did you feel like the diagnosis was right? If it wasn't, why not?

What do you wish you could tell your practitioner about what your diagnoses or lack of diagnoses mean to you? Would you have this conversation with your practitioners? Why or why not?

Ableism

Before my diagnosis, I knew people with disabilities, but I didn't think of myself as able-bodied. I just didn't think about it. When I was diagnosed, I very much rejected the idea of being someone with a disability or a disabled person. I didn't like it, I didn't want to interact with other people in chairs, I didn't want to go to support groups. I thought, "That's not me."

It took time, but I became more comfortable with the idea of having a disability. I had to work through a lot of my own internalized ableism. I rejected the idea of disability because I was taught that disability was bad.

I started opening up to having friends in chairs. I found this group of people that have changed my life so much. To have people around that just get it, who I know I don't have to explain if I need to cancel plans, my body's just not working well that day, who understand the difficulties and the challenges that come with being a wheelchair user in a world that is not super-accessible. I went from not thinking about disability to rejecting it to really embracing it. I am now proud of my identity as a disabled person. It is just part of being a human.

Ableism is prejudice and discrimination against people who have a disability. It relies on the construct that people who are "healthy" or have certain abilities are superior to others. Ableism is embedded in how we were educated as children. Much of the focus in perfection-driven cultures is on being good, achieving, fixing, excelling, being the best—being a "productive member of society." We deeply absorb the message that we are only worth what we produce.

Internalized Ableism

Being different runs counter to societal norms. Our own internal ableism—when we are afraid to ask for help or don't want to or can't acknowledge our disability—can prevent us from getting adequate care, forming and growing relationships, and living our best lives. When people with long illness feel themselves in a flare, their instinct may be to push harder (stay at work later, or take on a caregiving role for others) rather than tend to their own needs.

There is no benefit to ableism. Here are some wise words from some people living with long illness and disability. Everyone we talked to brought up their own ableism or discomfort with seeing themselves as sick, regardless of whether or not they accepted that they have a long illness.

Early on, I was honestly scared of other patients; I didn't want to be like them. I was ableist is what it boiled down to. And I had no idea. I just hadn't confronted those issues at all. I didn't want to be sick, like them. I didn't want to stay sick. It was really scary to see people whose lives were ruined by illness. I didn't want to think that that could be me. And, frankly, I bought into some of the prejudice. I thought, "I'm sick for real, but I don't know about those other people, maybe they're just crazy." I lost out for feeling that way, for not confronting my ableism sooner than I did. I lost out because other patients, in many ways, have been so helpful in my illness in a way that my doctors were unable to be.

I was so determined to say that my disease didn't change me. I was ready to put it all behind me, to go back to school and continue with my life exactly as before. But illness did change me. It put me into heart failure. It left me weak, winded, and weary. What I didn't realize is that this change wasn't a bad thing. I was more empathetic, took more time to care for myself, and was a better friend. Ultimately, it didn't matter that my body needed more care.

Are You Disabled?

Most long illnesses fall under the definition of a disability. Almost everyone will temporarily or permanently experience disability during their lifetime. In the United States, the Americans with Disabilities Act (ADA) defines a disability as having a physical or mental impairment that limits one or more major life activities. This definition includes many types of illness and is intentionally broad so that it can provide protection against discrimination for the greatest number of people.

This book is also addressed to those anywhere on the full spectrum of long illness. You may identify as disabled, or you may not. For many people, referring to themselves as disabled is an important part of their identity. Others acknowledge that they meet the criteria for disability, but the label doesn't resonate for them. You choose what fits you. Just remember that you have rights and access to support that is ready for you when you need it.

I remember coming out of surgery and saying to the guy who was wheeling me into the recovery room that I had my mother there, so that I would have someone to take me home. And he was like, "Oh no, she's not going to be allowed in there because of Covid," and I said, "Well, they said that they would allow her because I have a disability." He said, "Don't say that you're disabled," and I was like, "But I am, and disability is not a bad word." Even in my half-conscious state I was trying to tell this guy who is bringing me into the recovery room that disability wasn't a bad word.

I think a big part of the reason why some people do not consider certain conditions as a disability mainly has to do with ableism, and the idea that having something be a disability is inherently a bad thing. When I first was diagnosed with my condition, I did not identify with disability at all. In retrospect, I think it definitely had a lot more to do with ingrained ableism than it had to do with my condition.

Invisible Disability

Invisible disabilities, or "hidden" disabilities, are those that you are experiencing but that cannot be seen by others. If you have an invisible disability, you have a right to high-quality care and accommodations. Unfortunately, this does not always happen. People looking at you from the outside presume that they know what is happening inside of you. They often say things like, "You don't look sick," or "You look fine to me." These statements can be well intentioned, but end up feeling invalidating. Suffering worsens when it goes unseen.

Some people with invisible disabilities suffer alone and experience repeated invalidation from their communities and medical practitioners. This doesn't have to be your reality. Finding your community can be an empowering way to understand resources for your illness and what you may be entitled to.

Legislated Support for People with Long Illness

Many countries, including the United States, have laws in place to protect people who have disabilities from discrimination. The Americans with Disabilities Act, which was passed in 1990, "prohibits discrimination on the basis of disability in employment, state and local government, public accommodations, commercial facilities, transportation, and telecommunications."[2] Even if you do not identify as disabled, the ADA provides support for you when you need it. The ADA has provided benefits that all Americans can take advantage of, including wider doorways; ramps and graded transitions from streets to sidewalks; increased signage; larger bathrooms, elevators, and ATMs; and water fountains, ticket machines, and sinks of different heights. Many of us have benefited from these accommodations at one time or another. Most importantly, the ADA allows a large part of our society to participate in the activities of life more fully. Family and friends can access more places, and workplaces and schools are more inclusive of people with differences.

The ADA prevents discrimination in employment and offers protections on the job, but we need to acknowledge that people who are sick tend to be burdened with more tasks they have to do just to manage their daily lives. Finding money for bills and treatments, getting time off for appointments and sick days, and the emotional toll of living a life outside of the norm are stresses that can pile up. Work requires energy that you might not have if you are dealing with a long illness. Although many workplaces may try to be supportive of people with disabilities and chronic conditions, ensuring that you get this support can be another source of stress.

Most larger workplaces have a disability accommodation office through which you can request accommodations at work. Legally, information about these accommodations is kept private, although some accommodations are obvious and can make you feel exposed at work. Accommodations can be as simple as a comfortable chair, longer breaks, or being able to sit down when others have to stand. More complex requests might take longer to implement. In the United States, you do not have to disclose your diagnosis.

I had just been diagnosed a few years before I started a difficult job, and I was terrified I was going to get fired. I thought if anyone knew about my illness that they would think I wouldn't be able to do my job or that I couldn't keep up. Initially, I didn't tell anyone but a close friend. I overstressed myself trying to overcompensate at work and ended up hospitalized. I had to tell my boss. Luckily, I was able to get the accommodations I needed, which has been much better for my health.

Early in my illness, I didn't want to talk about it. I didn't want people to pigeonhole me. I didn't want people making accommodations because I was still in denial. I thought, "This isn't me, this doesn't define me," which, of course, it doesn't. But that way of dealing with my illness, by saying it doesn't define me, was just denying it was a part of my life. Being forced to deal with my illness at work was hard, but it led me to be more accepting of illness and pushed me to take better care of myself.

The Power of Community

Being involved in your community, whether by having a job or serving in the community in another role, can be beneficial for your health. Not only do people with long illness benefit from participating in their community, but so does society at large.

There are lots of different ways to get involved. In the United States, people receiving Social Security disability benefits can enroll in free and voluntary programs that will help them join and succeed in the workforce.[3] Besides a traditional job, other ways to participate in your community that give life meaning include making art, working in a community garden, being a supportive person to your friends, or helping your neighbors.

The chance that everyone you work with is going to be your ally is slim. Those of you who can work have probably experienced work-related stress around your condition. Some of you can't do shift work or work a demanding career job right now. If you live in a culture and tradition that sees serving the community as a vocation, the concept of "work" may be less of a priority for you. Activities that decrease isolation and loneliness in yourself and in others go a long way in contributing to the health of society, and to your own health.

Building Your Illness Community

The illness community as a whole has an incredible depth of knowledge about living with illness. Talking about relationship dynamics with caregivers, setting boundaries relating to my illness, these are conversations you just can't have outside of the patient community. Being able to talk to people who have a sense of what you are going through is invaluable. It's just a complete waste if you don't take advantage of that.

When I found a community of people who also don't always feel great, it gave me some perspective. I stepped back and realized that I was looking at my experiences with illness in a really negative light. I would think things like "I am so annoyed I can't do this or that I feel this way." I would fixate on my limitations. In talking to other people I realized that this illness has made me better at my job and a better human being. Before having a community with other people, I don't think I had ever looked at my illness as a strength.

Engaging in illness and disability communities can provide you with extra layers of support and allow you to share your hard-earned knowledge with others who are struggling. Ask your practitioners or visit websites about your conditions to find reputable support groups, read discussion threads, and connect with other people. Social workers or case managers at your primary care or specialists' offices have information on illness groups and ways to get involved in your community. If you join illness or disability visibility groups at work or at school, you'll see that allies are usually welcomed in those places too.

Your health care team can be a great source of strength, but they are not going to be able to be everything for you. Fortunately, having friends or acquaintances you can talk to about what you are going through can be life-changing. These allies might not be who you think they would be. You may often find yourself bonding with people who do not have your same illness, people who are not the same age as you, or even people with whom you have no common interests. Someone else with a long illness may be there for you. We have worked with many people who have found friends and lifesaving support by connecting with a community. It doesn't happen overnight, but with time you will find such a community too.

The families and friends of people who have long illness need support too. Encourage your family and caregivers to join caregiver support groups to learn more about what it means to be in their new role. Therapy and support are important, as the caregiver role is challenging and different from many other roles we take on in our lives.

Exercise: Who Can Provide Support?

There are ways in which you show support for people around you without even knowing it. A friendly wave, helping a neighbor carry groceries, letting another car pass you in traffic, or complimenting someone. These interactions build us up. Sometimes you need more than just kindness. You may need someone to advocate on your behalf, to drive you to an appointment, to wait with you for results, or to let you complain about a situation without judgment. It is important to acknowledge the people who give you support in living with a long illness, to appreciate these relationships, and to make sure they know how important they are to you. When you feel strong, you can provide support to them as well.

Tiny or huge, all contributions make a big difference. In your journal, jot down the names of the people who have given you support recently:

At home
At work
While doing hobbies or other activities
In your friend group
In your neighborhood
Online
In other ways

Any surprises while making this list?

If you were discouraged when thinking about who has given you support, you are not alone. We live in a disconnected world, one where loneliness is a public health concern. Some of you may realize that you don't have many people in your life who can provide deep levels of support. This is a common experience, but it's possible to find additional support. See the resources section at the back of the book for ideas on how to grow your own support community.

CHAPTER 3

Building Your Support System and Medical Team

Support from family, friends, others who have long illness, and groups is important. In the same way that you choose your support team, you will want to choose your medical team. There is a lot of jargon to take in when you get a diagnosis, as well as a never-ending list of health care practitioners who are now involved in your life. There are a lot of players in the game of health, and many of your practitioners might not be familiar with all that is out there.

What You Will Learn in This Chapter:

- The essential members of your health care team
- How to work with your primary care practitioner
- Tips for finding the best team members for you and your illness

What Is a Practitioner?

Throughout this book we use the word *practitioner* to be inclusive, as some people do not think of the main person on their health care team as a biomedical practitioner. When we use the word "practitioner" we usually are referring to a primary care practitioner in the biomedical model (physician, nurse-practitioner, physician's assistant). However, other types of practitioners might be able to answer your questions, and in some cases they can give you better answers than some biomedical practitioners.

More broadly, a practitioner is anyone with specialized education or training in the health sciences who interacts directly with people who have health needs. Listed here are some different practitioner types. Which of them have you worked with? Is there a type of practitioner we didn't list here who is important in your life?

Nurse	Dietitian	Physical therapist	Feldsher
Psychologist	Pharmacist	Midwife	Shaman
Medical assistant	Sangoma	Respiratory therapist	Dentist
Herbalist	Reiki teacher	Acupuncturist	Care assistant
Chiropractor	Surgeon	Physician	Medicine man
Curandero	Athletic trainer	Podiatrist	Tohunga
Aesthetician	Ayurvedist	Nganga	Osteopath
Optometrist	Chaplain	Nurse-practitioner	Physician's assistant
Nutritionist	Paramedic	Social worker	Occupational therapist
Speech and language pathologist		Doctor of Asian medicine	

Whoever you choose to see, you are two humans coming together. When you enter the room (virtually or in person), you arrive on equal footing. You are in control of what you discuss and what treatment you choose. You can ask to pause the visit or take a short break at any time. If you aren't feeling heard or understood, consider discussing this with the practitioner, if you feel safe doing so. If you don't, see if someone else is available who can meet your needs.

Your Primary Care Practitioner and Specialists

If you have a long illness, having a biomedical primary care practitioner is necessary for gaining access to most care. Depending on where you live and your health care coverage, you will be assigned to or choose a primary care practitioner, usually a physician, physician's assistant, or nurse-practitioner; that practitioner will serve as the base of your care team. For most of us, getting a primary care practitioner is luck of the draw. If you don't end up with a practitioner you like, see the next section, "What If You Aren't Clicking with Your Practitioner?," for tips on how to talk to the practitioner directly about how you can improve your relationship. If that doesn't work, see our advice on how to switch practitioners.

Many people are seen by a group of primary care practitioners, an arrangement that some of us find frustrating. You might not get to see your usual practitioner if you are coming in for an urgent visit. Let the staff and the practitioner know how important it is for you to see the same practitioner; also let them know if it's okay with you to see any of the practitioners. Practitioners take leave, move, and take new jobs, and sometimes that change is really difficult for patients. But if you are being seen by multiple practitioners at a primary care clinic, that could present opportunities for someone else to pick up on something about your illness or care that might have been overlooked, for you to find other practitioners you like, or for you to appreciate your primary practitioner more. As practitioners, we wish we could always see you when you come in, but that's just not how it works at most practices.

For some people with more complex long illnesses, specialists might serve as a second primary care doctor. For example, an obstetrician if you're pregnant, a rheumatologist if you have rheumatoid arthritis, or an oncologist if you're being treated for cancer might be more familiar with the ins and outs of your particular condition. Usually, a specialist communicates with your primary care practitioner and sometimes takes over some parts of your care that are more complicated and nuanced in your condition, such as administering treatments that a primary practitioner might not know or be able to prescribe or recommend.

Mutual respect between you and the practitioner is required for this relationship to be beneficial. If you feel like the practitioner is not listening, respecting your decisions, answering your questions, or making you feel safe and comfortable, it might be time to talk to this person about your concerns. Even if you do move on to a different practitioner, or plan to leave regardless of the outcome of your conversation, it is an opportunity for both of you to learn, and you might be surprised by what a positive experience it turns out to be.

Journaling

WORKING BETTER WITH YOUR PRIMARY CARE PRACTITIONER

Do you have a primary care practitioner?

What is your primary care practitioner like?

What do they do that you like?

What do you wish they could do differently?

Would you feel comfortable telling your primary care practitioner the thoughts that came to mind while journaling?

If there is something that your practitioner could do better, you can and should talk to them about it. Practitioners can take feedback, and most will try to deliver better care. Try sharing your thoughts with your practitioner at the next visit. If you don't feel comfortable doing so, consider why that may be and if that means you should change practitioners.

What If You Aren't Clicking with Your Practitioner?

Even though it might not seem like it all the time, most people get into health care because they want to help people. They want to do a good job. That said, we are all human. You may click with some practitioners more than others. Practitioners are aware that this is an issue, so bring it up.

It may seem scary, but just rip the Band-Aid off and say how you are feeling. There are many ways to do this. Don't be angry, and don't blame. Just give your practitioner the benefit of the doubt and lay it out there. Here's an example:

I feel like we need to take a step back here and look at the big picture. I do not feel like I am being heard. Can we pause and make sure we are on the same page? I want to feel better, and I want us to have a good relationship. I want you to be a person I can trust and that I want to reach out to when I need you.

If a practitioner doesn't respond well to being told that your needs are not being met, here are some other options:

Ask if there is another practitioner in the office you can see.

Call your insurance to see if you can visit a different office.

Ask if you can get a second opinion.

Ask to talk to the patient liaison or nurse manager, who are helpful with communication issues.

Talk to people in support groups or your medical communities to see if they have recommendations on alternative practitioners.

When you've fallen through the cracks before, you know the only way to get what you need is to advocate for yourself.

As a child, I was taught that doctors are the last word; you do what doctors say. Then I grew up and my roommate was a doctor. I got to see that doctors were indeed real humans, they could be wrong, they have personalities and feelings. I got more confident about being able to disagree, say what was important to me, and firing doctors and finding someone who was a better match for me. Eventually I found a care team for myself that I didn't necessarily always agree with, but that I believe in and that have my best interest in mind.

Other Practitioners to Find Before You Need Them

Your primary care practitioner will be just that: primary. But you may need others along the way. We recommend assembling this team early so that when you do need them, you don't have to scramble.

Mental health practitioner: Long illnesses take a psychological toll. A therapist and psychiatrist can be essential members of your care team. Building a relationship with someone takes time and it is helpful to build this relationship before you are in crisis. Establishing a few visits with a practitioner while you are well is a great way to have a resource in the community you can return to when you need it.

Establishing this relationship is easier said than done for most people, however, as access to mental health care is more limited than ever before. Some insurances don't cover therapy, and there can be long wait-lists. There are many different types of people who can provide mental support services, including licensed counselors, social workers, and people with PhDs or PsyDs in psychology. You may even find counseling through religious groups, community-based group therapy, or online groups. There are different styles and types of therapists, many of which are explored in our mental health chapters. Many people also find help through support groups, which are often free or low-cost and that focus on different things, from your type of illness to topics such as loss or pain.

TIPS

How to Find a Therapist

- Try a resource like psychologytoday.com to search for a therapist in your area who accepts insurance or sliding-scale fees (typically based on income).
- A call to your insurance company can help you with in-network referrals and in understanding out-of-pocket costs for seeing out-of-network practitioners.
- Local graduate school programs for various degrees often have therapists available at a discounted rate.
- Check with community centers and illness organizations to see if there are funds available to you for therapy.
- Consider support groups and group therapy to find pathways to individualized therapy.
- Ask your practitioner's office if they have an embedded therapist or someone on their staff who can help you connect with a therapist.

Dentist: Most people should go to their dentist twice a year for cleaning. If dental care is covered by your insurance, make an appointment today. Many people with a long illness are more susceptible to dental issues. Your dentist can keep an eye on your mouth so that you don't develop dental problems that add to your medical issues. Your dentist is also an incredible resource and might have some ideas about how to treat symptoms such as dry mouth, jaw pain, teeth grinding, and even sinus issues and headaches.

Vision professional: You should get your eyes checked yearly, or at least every few years. You can go to an optometrist, who tests how well you see and can diagnose and treat some eye conditions. Keeping your vision corrected can help with many symptoms, including headaches, nausea, dizziness, concentration, and fatigue. Depending on your underlying diagnosis and the medications you take, you might need to get support from an ophthalmologist, a physician who specializes in eye health. Your primary care practitioner, specialist, or optometrist can tell you if you need to go to an ophthalmologist.

Pharmacist: If you are getting medications filled near your home or work, get to know your local pharmacists. They are experts on medications and can often answer questions about side effects and interactions that your doctor may not be able to answer. If you have issues with insurance or approval for medication, it can be really helpful to have someone on your side.

TIPS

- Know where the twenty-four-hour pharmacies are near you.
- If your pharmacy has an app, download it and use it to make sure you are getting your refills on time. Set up automatic refills.
- If using mail services or pill packs might help you take your medication, ask your pharmacist about the best way to set up these services.
- Ask if there are any coupons or manufacturers' programs for your medications that aren't completely covered by insurance.

Long Illness After Hours

Let's say it's 2:00 a.m. and you are having a health crisis. What do you do when the health care practitioner's office is closed? What if going to the emergency room or a hospital would make things worse? Those hours or days spent waiting to get in touch with your primary team can be nerve-wracking.

We recommend that you talk to your primary care practitioner and other practitioners ahead of time about what to do if you have issues outside of regular hours. Most practitioners will give you a summary of your visit with information about who to call after hours, and many offices have after-hour help lines that you can use. Today those with electronic medical records can often access their own medical record online, which includes instructions for after-hours help. Put that number into your phone, just in case.

TIPS

Ask your practitioner:
- Is there anything that should not be given to me in the emergency room?
- Is there anything you would want to be called for in the middle of the night? (Many oncologists and practitioners who provide very specialized treatments prefer that their office be paged at night so that they can advise overnight practitioners.)

Insurance

If you do not have insurance, you should look into the health care exchanges and see what you qualify for. If your illness affects your ability to work and you have limited income and resources, you might be able to qualify for Medicaid or Medicare. There are many people who are not eligible for Medicaid yet cannot afford insurance on the exchanges, or don't want to pay for it. If you have a long illness, we advise you to get some type of insurance.

Insurance is far from perfect, but it can protect you from some debt and enable you to get preventative care and emergency care.

What is covered varies greatly by plan. Even if a particular treatment or service is covered by your insurance, the company might find a reason to reject the claim, or require that you pay out of pocket for some part of it. Insurance can be incredibly frustrating and a large source of stress for anyone interacting with the health care system. It is inevitable that those with long illness will be mischarged, denied coverage for covered needs, and forced to deal with multiple billing issues. Lean on your support network to help you. If something about an encounter with your insurance company seems unfair or off, it probably is. Sometimes we don't have energy to fight every battle, but you should speak up to your practitioners if you are having issues. Sometimes social workers or case managers can work with you to reduce or eliminate at least some of these issues.

TIPS

- We recommend taking an afternoon to review your health insurance, what it covers, and other options you might have to ensure that you have the best plan to cover your needs.
- If treatments you want to try are not covered, you can usually use money from a health savings account (HSA) or a flexible spending account (FSA). You are allowed to use pretax dollars from these accounts for approved health care expenses in the United States. (Note that you generally have to sign up for these during the initial enrollment period, or "open enrollment," which is mid-November through mid-December.)
- Many practitioners offer a cash discount or have sliding-scale fees.
- If you think there's been an error with an insurance claim, contact your practitioner. Sometimes you were turned down because your practitioner picked the wrong code, or because only a certain type of practitioner could order the treatment or service. Always ask.
- Tap your illness community for recommendations on cheap and free resources for exercise, nutrition, health care apps, and ways to be

approved for coverage by your particular insurance. It is an exhausting game, but other people have been playing it for a long time, so ask the community. They are a wealth of information on how to get treatments and services covered.

EXERCISE

YOUR MEDICAL TEAM

Using the list provided here, assemble info on all your relevant contacts. Keep it on your phone, and print it out as well. You may want to share this info with your family or friends.

If you can't fill in all of the info requested, use this list as a reminder to look it up or to keep looking for a type of practitioner you may not have found yet. You can also use the list to show you the appointments you should make next. Any info requested that's not relevant to you can be skipped. You can also add info that is more appropriate for you.

You can copy this list into your journal, or you can copy or scan and print out the form we provide in the resources section in the back of the book. Take a picture of it after you have filled it out and make it a favorite in your phone. Be sure to update the list when things change.

The basics: Name, contact information, notes

Insurance: Phone number, address, group and member numbers, and any other info that could be helpful, such as the number for a case manager at your insurance provider

Pharmacy: Phone number, address, and hours; also the phone number for the closest twenty-four-hour pharmacy

Primary practitioner: Most commonly, the phone number, address, and hours for the biomedical practitioner through whom you can access the conventional biomedical system

Emergency contact: Who should be called first if something happens to you? Does this person have a way to get in contact with other people you care about?

Medical decision-maker: If you are unable to make decisions about your care, who do you want to make those decisions for you? Think carefully

about this and make sure you choose someone who will make the decisions that you would make for yourself, not what they want for you or
want for themselves. This person might not be the same as your emergency contact.

Other practitioners: *Name, contact info, notes (last visit, next visit?)
for your therapist, dentist, optometrist or ophthalmologist, specialists,
physical or occupational therapist, and other practitioners*

TIP

Save pictures of your insurance cards, back and front, as favorites in your
phone as well as a picture of your photo ID. You will be asked for these
often.

PART II

COMMON SYMPTOMS

When a symptom comes up for the first time, it can be hard to know where to turn. You may ask yourself, "Should I be worried? How is this treated?" For symptoms that have persisted over months or years, you may wonder if there's more that could be done, or whether you have the right diagnosis. Are there supplements you should try? How will you ever feel better?

The following chapters are a comprehensive resource you can use to navigate the most common symptoms of long illness. We explain the physiology behind each symptom, describe workup and treatment, and arm you with tools to add to your healing tool kit.

We start with the primary reason people seek care: pain. Then we cover fatigue and the most common neurologic symptoms: brain fog, dysautonomia, and headache. We end with breathing problems, digestion, and sleep.

In these chapters, we give you information and tools for managing the most common complaints we treat. Feel free to skip to the symptom that plagues you the most. Bring this book with you to your next appointment to explore more options for treatment. We use our favorite recipe for healing: knowledge, support, and tools.

CHAPTER 4

Pain

I try to never use the "P" word or ask for painkillers. I have learned to wait for my doctors to offer them, so that they will think I am a good patient. I decline when offered an opioid: "Oh no, I would never want to take that." I praise my doctors, telling them how smart and good they are, how they have helped me, all while suffering in pain, praying that they will have anything to offer me.

While pain is gone, I am free. When I think about the pain, I say, "It wasn't that bad," "Maybe it was from this or that," "That will never happen again," "Next time I will just...." Maybe it's denial. I don't know. But then, one day, just as suddenly as it left, pain comes back. I throw everything I have at it, hoping I can avoid doctors. I hope that my plan for supplements, painkillers, heating pads, exercise, rest, baths, using sick days, meditating, and deep breathing will work this time.

What You Will Learn in This Chapter:

- Common types of pain and reasons for pain in long illness
- The full spectrum of treatment options for pain, including nonpharmacologic approaches, medications, procedures, and natural products
- How to build your own personalized pain tool kit

Pain is the most common reason people seek medical care. This is true for most of those with long illness as well. Pain interferes with the ability to work and participate in our communities. People with pain have a lower quality of life and face many kinds of stigma, including from their practitioners. Many pain sufferers end up feeling desperate, isolated, and frustrated.

Pain is difficult for many practitioners and health care systems to address. In addition, the misrepresentation of the safety of opioids by pharmaceutical companies has resulted in a worldwide health crisis during which many practitioners unintentionally promoted the misuse of opioids in our communities. The pendulum has now swung to the other extreme, with many practitioners undertreating pain, conducting involuntary tapers off opioids, or cutting patients off of opioids completely, increasing the risk that people will seek nonprescribed opioids outside of the medical setting. Many practitioners do not evaluate patients for an opioid use disorder (OUD), a very common side effect of chronic opioid use, and so do not offer any of the evidence-based therapies for OUD when indicated. Furthermore, many patients have endured stigma from medical practitioners who label them as "drug seeking."

If this is your story, either in whole or in part, we want you to know that we hear and see your pain and recognize the difficulties that many people have with pain and pain treatment.

At its simplest, acute pain is easy to diagnose and treat. Something inside or outside of the body (a *stimulus*) causes pain, and when the stimulus is removed, pain disappears. Pain that doesn't get better, or pain that comes back, is called *chronic pain*. Chronic pain is more common in long illness because the underlying stimulus (inflammation, damage) has not been removed or stopped. Some treatments might work for a while, but they may lose their effectiveness or become hard to access.

When you have an episode of acute pain, your body releases your own endogenous opioids to help ease it. This happens quickly and regularly. In chronic pain, however, the ability to tap into your endogenous opioids is diminished.

The landscape may seem bleak, but there is much hope to be had. The treatment of chronic pain can make changes in your brain that reverse pain-related changes. Preventative activities like exercise, meditation, and other activities that build your parasympathetic nervous system often act in a neuroprotective manner to prevent changes in the brain due to chronic pain.

Let's dive in and explore pain a little more and how it works. We will share some tools that can be helpful in dealing with pain and show you how to come up with a pain plan.

What Is Pain?

The International Association for the Study of Pain defines pain as an *unpleasant sensory and emotional experience* accompanied by actual or potential tissue damage, or your impression that there has been tissue damage. Pain protects you from your environment, giving you a signal that something is harmful to you, or could be. Almost everyone has experienced *acute pain*—that sudden pain that gets better after a few seconds, minutes, or weeks. Chronic pain is also common: about one out of every five people on earth has dealt with chronic pain in their lifetime.

Pain is not something you can simply fight through. The parts of your brain that interpret pain are closely connected to the parts of your brain that manage your attention and emotions, so experiencing pain impairs your attention and negatively affects your emotions.

We all experience pain differently based on many factors, including our cultural, spiritual, or learned experiences. Pain is stigmatized in many cultures as something we should be able to control or endure. People are often told to calm down or to focus on something else. Changes in attention and emotions, however, are symptoms of pain. What if you had an upset stomach and someone told you to stop throwing up? Would that help? The idea of ignoring pain is just as laughable as not vomiting when you have a stomach bug.

How Is Pain Different in People with Long Illness?

Your brain is built to learn and adapt. When you experience stress and trauma, your nervous system can become overactive and hypervigilant. If you have long illness, here are some experiences that can prime your nervous system to worsen your pain:

- Difficult or adverse childhood experiences (ACEs) that taught your brain to be overprotective and made you feel you might be in trouble even though you're currently safe
- Difficult experiences as an adult, such as loss of a job or a loved one, trauma, or changes in your environment
- Inadequate treatment of a preexisting condition, like depression and fibromyalgia, which already induces higher levels of pain, making it harder to manage pain well
- Everyday stress manifesting as physical symptoms, like headache, backache, or upset stomach, if you have an overactive nervous system
- Having personality traits or coping mechanisms, such as being a people-pleaser or perfectionist, that can keep your nervous system in a tense and vigilant state
- Increased amygdala (fear center) activity following threats to your health such as incorrect diagnoses, hospitalizations, surgeries, gaslighting, or negative interactions with practitioners, resulting in a more intense experience of pain that can create an exaggerated fear of pain (sometimes referred to as *pain catastrophizing*)
- Heightened pain from the isolation, worsening mental health, and decrease in social and physical activity that can result from living with long illness

When your pain is chronic and the neural pathways have been used over and over to let you know pain is there, the pathways get fast and efficient. They can overreact and tell you that you might be in pain soon, even if that is not the case. The more you experience pain, the stronger those connections are.

Describing Your Pain

Practitioners think about pain based on answers to four big questions: Where is it (location)? When did it start (duration)? What is the pain from (cause)? What is the pathophysiology (type) of the pain? This helps them think about the steps to take next to treat it. These questions also can help you learn to describe your pain in a language that your practitioner can more quickly understand.

There are four main types of pain that practitioners consider when thinking about treatments. You can have combinations of all of these.

Type	Source	Examples	What Helps	What It Feels Like
Nociceptive	Inflammation, tissue damage, somatic (localized, for example, in the leg) versus visceral (diffuse, for example, in an internal organ)	Broken leg, arthritis, bruise, burn	Treating underlying cause or stopping stimulus, anti-inflammatories, opioids (mainly for acute pain)	Stabbing, crushing, sharp, dull, aching, throbbing
Neuropathic	Nerve damage, though the body "appears normal"	Spinal cord injury, neuropathies, compression of nerve, drug side effects, bumping the "funny bone" (elbow)	Treating underlying cause, antidepressant medications, neuropathic pain agents	Pins and needles, numbness, itching, burning, coldness, electric-shock-like, shooting, stabbing, throbbing
Nociplastic/ central sensitization	Dysfunction in processing of pain signals	Chronic pain, fibromyalgia, chronic opioid use	Exercise, education, medications, physical therapy, psychotherapy, pain-targeting procedures, mind-body medicine, chiropractic care	Pain everywhere, or pain out of proportion to what is expected
Psychogenic	Mental, emotional, or behavioral factors in the absence of any physical indication of related disease	Headache, stomach pain, or back pain, usually after a major emotional event; common in childhood	Education, compassion, therapy	Can feel like any type of pain

Aside from describing the sensory experience of pain, perhaps the most important component of your pain story is *being able to describe the impact of the pain on your life*. Tell your practitioner if your sleep has changed, if you have stopped showering or getting dressed for the day, if you are avoiding people or situations, or if you are withdrawing from life. Pain treatment works best with a team of practitioners who know you well (see Chapter 3 on building your medical team).

Building Your Pain Management Tool Kit

People experience pain differently. One headache might not feel exactly like another, even in the same person. A treatment you have used forever might stop working. With pain it is best to prepare a multimodal plan for when pain is difficult to manage. Remember that pain interferes with your ability to concentrate, so having a plan ready can be helpful to ensure that you're able to address your pain quickly.

If you're interested in any of the common pain therapies outlined here, we suggest discussing them with your practitioners. Besides prescribing and recommending medications based on your health history, they can provide you with resources and referrals.

Our list of pain therapies is not exhaustive. Our intention in compiling this list is to let you know that there are a lot of interventions for pain and different specialists who can help you address it. While reading through the list, take notes on which treatments have worked for you in the past and in what situations they were helpful. Even if you have tried a particular therapy before and it didn't help, keep an open mind. It might be useful in the future, even for the same issue. These notes will help you build your plan at the end of the chapter.

Nonpharmacologic Therapies: "Distract and Decrease"

Nonpharmacologic therapies should be your go-to, first-line therapies for the prevention and treatment of pain. They are generally low-risk, free or low-cost, and accessible. These methods all work in different ways. Some of them distract the brain from the pain signal and divert the attention to the new stimulus you provide. Some methods work to increase the release of your own natural supply of pain medication, called *endorphins*, resulting in hours of pain relief.

Evidence for the efficacy of some of these methods is strong. Evidence supporting some others is limited, but because they are unlikely to be harmful, we have included all of them for you to consider trying. A recent large study found that mind-body therapies (meditation, hypnosis, relaxation, guided imagery, therapeutic suggestion, cognitive behavioral therapy) improve pain and can lower the use of medications.

Since medications and procedures to control pain often fall short when used alone, we need more in our tool kits. It can be frustrating to be offered treatment options that you probably tried early in your experience of pain and that fell short. But even a 5 percent reduction in pain can increase functioning. When we weave nonpharmacologic therapies into your existing pain plan, there can be noticeable results. Harnessing the power of these tools can be important in preventing and decreasing pain.

Ice/cold compress	Great for inflammatory or myofascial (muscle and the support tissue surrounding it) pain. If you feel aching, tight, pulling, deep, or boring pain, especially in your neck and shoulders or major joints, cold might help.
Heat/heating pad	Our first go-to for myofascial pain. Helps loosen muscles. Use heat before self-massage. Ice after might be helpful for some.
Deep breathing	Most of us do this automatically to calm ourselves. Deep breathing can reboot an overexcited nervous system. Focusing on breathing makes it easier to relax. Regular practice can help you calm and center yourself more quickly when stressed.
Getting comfortable/ ergonomics	If you are in pain from doing a daily task (using a computer, using your hands), stop, step back, and reevaluate. Simply changing positions may relieve the pain. Set yourself up to avoid pain by taking breaks, making modifications in your work setup, and stopping to rest when you first feel discomfort. When you are in pain, stop and get into a comfortable, safe environment.

Calm environment	Unpleasant sensory input, including loud or annoying sounds, strong smells, or intense lighting, can exacerbate pain. At home or in other places where you spend a lot of time, go to a dark, quiet, smell-free nook where you can turn down your sensory intake.
Nature	Spending time in nature can help with pain tolerance by decreasing stress and anxiety and boosting mood. Just looking at pictures of nature can decrease your perception of pain, lessen your anxiety, and increase your tolerance of pain. Nature sounds can decrease stress and pain.
Bathing	Baths are relaxing, and they can increase circulation and ease the pain of sore muscles. Immersion, buoyancy, and vibration are all novel sensory inputs into your nervous system that can inhibit pain signals.
Self-massage	Any type of self-massage can be soothing to the nervous system. Using an oil can provide feedback to the nervous system and make it easier to massage. You can use tennis balls or a Thera Cane to do trigger-point massage (using heat before and ice after).
Self-acupressure	Go online to find out about different points on your body to practice on, or ask an acupuncturist, massage therapist, or physical therapist to teach you a few.
Guided imagery/ visualization	Guided imagery or visualization transports you to a more relaxed state in which you can imagine yourself in a more comfortable situation. It can help reduce your perception of pain and increase your pain tolerance.
Meditation/mindfulness	Routine meditation or meditation during pain crises can decrease pain, protect against neuroanatomical changes in the nervous system, decrease symptoms of depression, and increase quality of life. Mindfulness-based pain management classes are available and might be covered by your insurance or recommended by your practitioner.
Spirituality/prayer	Prayer is a type of concentration or meditation. Like meditation, it can reduce stress and pain.
Snacks	Being hungry increases cortisol levels and can increase your sensation of pain. Eating a healthy snack can decrease pain.
Exercise	Daily movement helps decrease inflammation, maintains or improves function, prevents deconditioning, improves blood flow, and can reduce pain and pain flares.
Tai chi	Tai chi improves quality of life, decreases pain, and relieves stiffness from various types of joint pain and pain from fibromyalgia.
Yoga	Yoga increases flexibility and range of motion and has the same effect on pain and disability as exercise or physical therapy.

Feldenkrais	This is a technique whose goal is to integrate mind and body through movement. Like similar techniques (for example, the Alexander technique), Feldenkrais can provide you with insight about how you use your body and how this contributes to your pain. The movements provide your brain with feedback and allow for neuroplasticity so that you can change your movement patterns. Feldenkrais, which is practiced mostly on the floor, is accessible to many people because it involves slow, small movements. You can practice it at home, in a class, or one-on-one with a practitioner facilitating your movements. This method can decrease pain, increase quality of life and body awareness, and decrease disability.
Talking to others	Being heard and having your experience validated by someone else can reduce your pain and stress. Also, listening to a friend tell a story can distract you and help you focus your attention away from your pain.
Expectation of relief/ placebo effect	If you expect relief from a treatment, your body responds by releasing its own, naturally synthesized opioids, even if you know that you are getting a placebo treatment.

A Note on the Placebo Effect

Many people use "placebo" like it's a bad word, believing that the relief you think it brings is all in your head and not real. But the placebo effect is very real. You get a natural opioid release with a placebo. It is so real that giving people naloxone (a medication that blocks opioids) blocks the placebo effect. Our brain has a system in place that we can hijack to give ourselves power over our own pain. So much power, in fact, that even knowing the placebo will not work but believing that it will, we get the release of endogenous stores of opioids and feel better. It's a measurable effect, which is why, when researchers test drugs, they test against a placebo.

Nonpharmacologic Therapies: Devices and Interventions

Like nonpharmacologic therapies, therapeutic devices and interventions cause minimal to no harm. Because they involve a device or another person or practitioner, they tend to require more energy to access. You have to buy a device and learn to use it. You have to schedule appointments and travel to appointments, and sometimes these treatments are not covered by insurance. Refer to Chapter 3 on building your medical team for more on how to handle these situations.

TENS unit	Transcutaneous electrical nerve stimulation (TENS) units are small devices that connect to your skin with sticky pads and deliver an electrical signal that can inhibit and reduce pain signals. TENS units can be helpful in treating chronic musculoskeletal pain (like low back pain), osteoarthritis pain, postoperative pain, neuropathic pain, and fibromyalgia. They are relatively inexpensive and can be bought at a drugstore without a prescription, or you can try them out at physical therapy.
Massage device	Home massage devices can provide distraction from pain. A recent study on mice in which a simulation of the popular massage gun was administered showed that the device decreased inflammation.
Massage	Not only does massage feel good, but it increases circulation and relaxation, which can decrease inflammation as well as reduce pain.
Physical therapy (PT)	PT evaluation can help you address the impact of chronic pain on your ability to move and participate in physical activities. Both physical therapists and occupational therapists prescribe exercises or devices that can help reduce pain.
Occupational therapy (OT)	An occupational therapist evaluates the impact of pain on your ability to work, take care of yourself, sleep, and interact with your family. An OT can help you pace and adapt the meaningful activities in your life so that you complete them.
Acupuncture	Acupuncture is effective in the treatment of chronic musculoskeletal pain, headache, arthritis pain, and other pain. For more on acupuncture, see Chapter 20 on traditional medicine.
Biofeedback	This technique teaches you how to recognize clues that your body is stressed out, like an increase in your heart rate and changes in muscle tension. It can decrease stress and increase parasympathetic tone, and practicing it can prevent pain during procedures. Biofeedback is effective at reducing headache pain as well as other types of pain.
Chiropractic manipulation	Chiropractic care is as effective as physical therapy for reducing low back pain and reducing chronic neck pain and improving function. Including chiropractic care in a multimodal approach to chronic pain, rather than chiropractic care alone, has better results.

Therapy	Cognitive behavioral therapy (CBT), which has been well studied, helps reduce pain, disability, and distress in chronic pain. Also studied has been acceptance and commitment therapy (ACT), which has shown no significant differences in pain and quality of life but does increase the ability to function and decrease anxiety and depression.
Hypnosis	Either self-hypnosis or hypnosis with a trained practitioner can reduce pain and improve your quality of life. And don't worry, no one will make you cluck like a chicken. Therapeutic hypnosis is not exactly what you have seen on TV.
Reiki/therapeutic touch	From East Asian medicine, Reiki, an energy healing technique, can decrease pain, anxiety, and depression and improve your quality of life through gentle touch. Therapeutic touch, a similar modality, also has been shown to decrease pain and improve quality of life.

Pharmacological Therapies: Supplements, Natural Products, and Over-the-Counter Drugs

Mild deficiencies in certain vitamins and minerals can cause or worsen pain. There is evidence that ensuring that people with chronic pain have appropriate levels of vitamin D, magnesium, iron, and B_{12} can prevent and treat some aspects of their pain. You can ask your practitioner to test your levels of the minerals and vitamins listed here. We have included the optimal levels and supplements that may help.

There are many supplements that treat pain. We have included information about a few of them in this list. Use the resources provided in Chapter 21 as well as by your care team and community to decide if something is right for you. Increasing your consumption of foods that are high in antioxidants and have anti-inflammatory properties can help with inflammation and oxidative stress, which are higher in people experiencing pain. As always, before you start any supplements or natural products, be sure to consult with your practitioner to make sure they're right for you and that there are no contraindications with medications you may be taking.

Magnesium	With magnesium, blood tests aren't the most reliable indicators of deficiency, but they're not needed for small-dose supplementation if your kidneys are healthy. Magnesium is often recommended for many pain syndromes. Magnesium glycinate is a formulation that crosses the blood-brain barrier with relative ease, and it does not usually cause GI upset. Consider discussing with your care team whether you should take 200–400 milligrams (ml) of magnesium twice daily. The optimal level is more than 2.2 milliequivalents per liter (mEq/L).
Vitamin B_{12}	Neurological dysregulation can begin at B_{12} levels as low as 400 milligrams. Taking 1,000 micrograms (ug) of oral B_{12} daily for a few months with retesting is recommended if B_{12} is low. The oral formulation is as effective as injected B_{12} for most people.
Iron	Ferritin, a marker of iron stores, can be elevated in people with long illness. A practitioner will usually test your iron saturation level. Using these levels, you can decide with your practitioner whether adding oral iron might be useful. Oral iron is constipating to many, and some studies have shown the same benefit from taking oral iron every other day rather than daily. Try to take iron with vitamin C and on an empty stomach, as that helps with absorption. Some people need IV iron, which can be helpful, especially when GI bleeding or heavy menses has caused significant blood loss. Iron supplementation is sometimes the only treatment needed for people experiencing the pain from restless leg syndrome.
Vitamin D	Supplementation of vitamin D in people with chronic pain can reduce pain levels and improve sleep as well as various aspects of quality of life. Taking 1,000–2,000 vitamin D units daily can be continued indefinitely, but high-dose supplementation over the long term is not advised.
Acetaminophen/ paracetamol	Conditions that improve with acetaminophen are limited; they include knee or hip osteoarthritis, migraine, tension headache, perineal pain after childbirth, and kidney stones. There is no evidence that taking it daily for chronic pain is helpful. Because acetaminophen should be avoided or reduced in dose for people with liver disease and overdoses can be lethal owing to liver damage, be sure to talk to your practitioner about whether acetaminophen is safe for you. This medicine is included in many cold and flu medications, so you might be taking more acetaminophen than you think. Take with caution.
NSAIDs	Nonsteroidal anti-inflammatory drugs (NSAIDs) like ibuprofen, aspirin, or naproxen sodium are highly effective medications that decrease inflammation. Talk to your practitioner about whether they are safe for you. Some people with kidney disease, cardiovascular risk factors, or GI disease, as well as those on blood thinners or medications that impact the kidneys, might need to avoid these medications or learn more about when and how to use them. If you find yourself overusing them, talk to your health care practitioner. NSAIDs have their place, but they can cause issues if used long-term.

Capsaicin	Derived from chili peppers, capsaicin is an irritant that is applied as a cream or gel to a local area of pain to distract the nervous system from the initial pain signal. Recently, higher-dose prescription patches have become available.
Lidocaine, topical	Applied to areas of pain as a patch, cream, or gel, lidocaine blocks sodium channels and can decrease pain signals. Lidocaine is usually inexpensive and covered by insurance. Patches are available over the counter.

Cannabis	There is not as much research on therapeutic uses of cannabis. Cannabis products should be obtained from regulated dispensaries, as cannabis from unknown sources can contain contaminants such as heavy metals or even other drugs. We break cannabis products down into two categories:
	
	    THC-containing cannabis products: Tetrahydrocannabinol is the psychoactive (intoxicating) compound in cannabis. When choosing a cannabis product for a long illness, it's important to know that cannabis products have a wide range of THC concentrations. Levels in research and medical cannabis are far below 10 percent, and amounts as low as 1 to 2 percent are enough to help manage pain. Cannabis products from recreational dispensaries average 13 percent THC, with concentrations in some products in the high 30s, although many dispensaries carry low-THC products. Higher THC does not bring more pain control. Higher THC concentrations also have more psychoactive effects, with potentially greater risks. Unfortunately, for older adults or people at higher risk for falls, THC-containing cannabis products can increase the risk of falls and injury. Paranoia, worsened concentration and memory, and anxiety are also common side effects. For some, THC-containing cannabis products are well tolerated. But we are still learning about long-term effects. Atrophy in the memory centers of the brain and lower cognitive scores have been found in long-term users of cannabis. The research is evolving daily, but current research suggests that using THC-containing cannabis for shorter periods of time is likely to be safer.
	
	    Other cannabinoids: There are more than 100 chemical components in cannabis that do not have psychoactive (intoxicating) effects, including cannabidiol (CBD) and cannabinol (CBN). Early research suggests that they may be beneficial in helping with pain; ongoing research is also studying their impact on anxiety and sleep. Many CBD/CBN products, even those sold over the counter, can have small amounts of THC; for example, hemp oil sold over the counter has a legal limit of 0.3 percent THC. CBD does not need THC to have benefits, but it may have more to offer when combined with THC-containing cannabis. In research thus far, CBD products generally have a good safety profile over the short term.
	
	Because of the potential risks of products containing higher concentrations of THC, we favor non-THC or low-THC products for our patients who find cannabis to be helpful. Like any herb, cannabis should be thought of as a medication, and its risks and benefits should be weighed with your health care team.

Pharmacological Therapy: Prescriptions and Interventions

We need better pain medication. Only 50 percent of people with chronic pain experience improvement with the available drugs, averaging 30 percent reduction in pain. That means that medications won't help half of you reading this who experience pain, and if you do, the reduction in your pain will usually be small. Also, these drugs have big-time side effects and can interact with other drugs you are taking. However, they may help some of you some of the time, so you should not be discouraged from trying them. If these drugs don't work, you can try different doses, routes, or timing, you can try again at a later time, or you can try them with a different practitioner guiding you. And if they do work for you, great! But keep in mind that for most people there is no single magic pill. And if you do find your magic pill, it may not work forever. That is why having a big tool kit of different things to try is key.

Pain medication works on nerves in different ways to decrease the signal of pain and increase the chemicals that can inhibit pain. Each of the drugs described here acts on a different part of the neuron to help reduce pain. Many of them were originally formulated for depression, anxiety, or seizures and were later found to also help people with pain. That is why some of them are called "antidepressants" or "anticonvulsants."

Many different neurochemicals play a role in pain signaling and local response to pain. Many of the prescribed medications increase or decrease the ability of the neurochemicals to signal, ideally resulting in a reduction in pain. Similarly, other drugs can stop electrical signals from being sent.

Here are some commonly prescribed medications:

Tricyclic antidepressants (TCAs)	TCAs are most often used for neuropathic pain and are also used to treat sleep disturbances and depression. They can interact with other drugs and should be used with caution in older adults and people with other medical conditions. Among the many different TCAs, the most commonly used are nortriptyline and amitriptyline.

Serotonin-norepinephrine reuptake inhibitors (SNRIs)	These medications improve both mood and pain. Selective serotonin reuptake inhibitors (SSRIs) have also been tried for pain, but they do not work as well as SNRIs. Duloxetine and venlafaxine are two commonly used SNRIs.
Anticonvulsants (ACs)	There are many different anticonvulsant medications; those used most often for pain are gabapentin and pregabalin.
N-methyl-D-aspartate (NMDA)–receptor blockers	Ketamine is the most commonly known NMDA-receptor blocker. While great in theory, this medication doesn't work as well for pain as was hoped. In addition, its potential for intense psychological dissociative and psychotic side effects limits its long-term use for pain.
Methadone	Methadone is best known as a treatment for people with opioid use disorder, but it is also a good treatment for chronic pain. Classified as an opiate, methadone acts quickly, lasts a long time, is cheap, and affects three different pain treatment pathways. Because of the societal stigma against people who use drugs, as well as legal limitations, many practitioners feel less comfortable prescribing this medication.
Buprenorphine	Buprenorphine has been used to treat people with opiate use disorder and is also used for treating chronic pain.
Naltrexone	Naltrexone is thought to work by reducing neuro-inflammation. It has been studied in chronic pain syndromes and shows promise in reducing symptoms for other complaints of long illness, including fatigue and brain fog, when used at low doses.
Opioids	Opioids[4] make you feel different fast. Many short- and long-term issues are associated with them, however, aside from development of an OUD. Naloxone can reverse the dangerously slow breathing that can lead to accidental death from overdose. Always request a prescription for naloxone (Narcan) so that you can keep it on hand in case you or someone else becomes too sedated (or "out of it") after taking opioids. Naloxone can be obtained with a prescription from a pharmacy, but it can also be found at harm-reduction sites or through local or national groups.[5] Prolonged use of opioids can lead to worse pain (opioid-caused hyperalgesia), immunosuppression, and hormonal changes.
Opioids for neuropathic pain	Tramadol and tapentadol are similar to an SNRI. If you are trying opioid pain medication for neuropathic pain, these might be the best option. However, they still carry the same risks as other opioids.
Other pain medications	Baclofen, alpha-2 agonists (clonidine, dexmedetomidine), and cannabinoids (not THC) are just some of the less commonly used drugs that have been studied for pain. If your practitioner suggests other drugs, ask what the studies say for people who are experiencing pain like yours.

Interventional Therapy

Interventional therapies require a specialized pain practitioner, usually a physician or surgeon trained in administering the specialty therapy.

Trigger point injections ("a shot to numb the pain") are superficial injections of lidocaine at trigger points that might be helpful if you are having myofascial pain. Joint and epidural injections bring steroids and numbing medication into a space to numb pain and reduce inflammation locally. These two procedures are commonly done by many types of practitioners. If your situation is more complicated, or your primary team is unable to do these types of interventions, you might be referred to a specialist.

Prolotherapy is a procedure in which an irritating substance is injected into a joint, with the goal of increasing the joint's stability and reducing overall inflammation upon healing.

Botox injections are used for the treatment of migraine headaches and can also be used to loosen tight muscles (like jaw muscles in those with temporomandibular joint (TMJ) disorder. These procedures are done by specialized pain doctors.

Transcranial magnetic stimulation uses magnets outside your body to change your brain patterns to reduce pain. It is helpful for chronic pain, but it can be expensive, is often not covered by insurance, and can require many visits to a practitioner to get an effect. A specialist should be consulted; psychiatrists have the most expertise in this field.

Nerve blocks, nerve ablation, peripheral nerve stimulators, and spinal cord neuromodulators are all interventions aimed at blocking nerve signals. In rare cases, a device commonly referred to as a "pain pump" can be implanted. Pain pumps infuse various types of medications into the nervous system directly via the spinal cord. There are significant risks associated with these devices. If you think that one of these therapies might be beneficial to you, discuss a referral to a pain physician with your primary practitioner.

Although some people do experience improvement with these interventions, they are not the first stop. They are often unsuccessful over the long term without a multimodal pain plan that focuses on nonpharmacologic work, like therapy and development of coping skills, and that uses pharmacological and interventional therapy only when necessary.

Journaling

BUILD YOUR TOOL KIT

In your journal, for each modality write down any treatments that have worked for you and also treatments described here that you might want to learn more about and try. You might have been treated in ways that fit into one or more of these categories, so also add your favorites to this list.

Nonpharmacologic therapies: Distract and decrease

Nonpharmacologic therapies: Devices and interventions

Pharmacological therapies: Supplements, natural products, and over-the-counter medications

Pharmacological therapies: Medications for which prescriptions are (usually) required

Interventional therapy

Example: Maria's endometriosis pain

Take a bath, nap, walk in nature. Want to try deep breathing.

Heating pad, massage. Want to try acupuncture.

Tylenol and ibuprofen. Want to learn more about my magnesium and vitamin D levels.

SNRI. Want to learn more about hormonal therapies, but have had bad experiences with birth control in the past.

Talking to my gynecologist about procedures that might be helpful.

When you have made your list, reflect on it and then share it with a friend, maybe someone who has seen you in pain or who spends a lot of time with you. This can spark a conversation about ways in which they can be helpful to you when you are in pain. Keeping this list is also handy when you are so overwhelmed that you forget what can make you feel better.

What Should You Do if Your Pain Flares?

Pain flares can be physically and emotionally devastating. We have found that a pain plan truly helps our patients in times of crisis. A pain plan outlines things that are helpful to have on hand, what others can do for you, and a decision tree of what steps to take. The plan takes the thinking out of what to do next. You want to come up with your pain plan when you are feeling good, and then add to it when you learn more about your pain.

A pain plan can be as simple as the list you just made. Some people find that writing out a plan for dealing with the next flare can be helpful. Write out your plan for the next time pain returns. Here is an example:

Hip Pain

Day 1:

   Self-care: Take it easy, heat a healthy soup for lunch, tell close friends
      about the pain flare

   Actions: Do gentle PT stretches, write in journal

   Pain control: Use heating pad and TENS unit for fifteen minutes, take
      a bath, wear hip support belt

   Other: Make PT appointment, schedule massage

Day 2:

   Self-care: Extra hydration, call in sick to work to rest

   Actions: Do gentle PT stretches, go for short walk to move body
      outdoors

   Pain control: Use heating pad and TENS unit for fifteen minutes, take
      a bath, wear hip support belt

   Other: Message primary care practitioner that I have started taking
      naproxen and ask if there is more I should be doing

Now make a pain plan for yourself. Think through what you will do the next time your pain flares. Making your plan while you are not in a crisis is helpful. You might discover that, when not in pain, you know exactly what to do when you are.

Why Are Opioids Not Recommended for Most Chronic Pain Conditions?

Chronic pain is unrelenting. Just when you think you have it under control, it can flare when you're injured or experience a stressor. You just want to make it go away. Opioids are great medications that make you feel different quickly. For short periods of time, they can be very useful in certain situations, such as when pain is greatly limiting your quality of life.

For chronic pain, however, there is no evidence that opioids are better than non-opioid pain medications. In fact, opioid prescriptions for chronic pain, compared to non-opioid prescriptions, are associated with an increased risk of all-cause mortality (not just deaths from overdose). Even for acute pain, studies have shown that people who are given an NSAID and acetaminophen have a pain experience similar to the pain experiences of those who receive an opioid and acetaminophen.

The goal of pain treatment is to maintain quality of life, to make life worth living. Any use of opioids, prescribed or not, puts you at risk for developing opioid use disorder, putting this treatment goal out of reach.

If you are prescribed opioids, ask your practitioner why you should take them and what the plan is for stopping their use. Make sure you have a follow-up visit soon after to talk about how your pain is doing so that you can stop as soon as possible. If you are prescribed opioids for longer-term use, you usually will have to sign a contract with your practitioner's office, for liability reasons. For some people, opioids may sometimes be the only thing that gets them through the day. If you fall into this category, we want to challenge you to continue to question your use of opioid pain medication. Try other therapies and occasionally try to taper off. It is essential to find other means of pain relief because not only does your body change, but the medication is dangerous and becoming harder and harder to legally obtain. Whether the legal complications are wrong or right is not the issue; we are making this recommendation because of the reality of the side effects both individual and societal. For some of you, opioids might be all that works right now. We hope that there eventually will be better medications you can try for the types of pain you are experiencing.

For those of you dealing with the stigma associated with opioid use, we hear you. Pain is a terrible situation to be in, and when you find something that seems to work, why would you ever want to stop it? Be honest with your practitioners about your concerns, and let them know if you're using more and more of the drug but it is no longer helping. It is worth exploring other ways of controlling your pain.

Why Is It Hard for Some Practitioners to Help You Address Your Pain?

We have all experienced pain, but many people have not experienced pain that makes them go to the emergency room and stops them from being able to function. There are many reasons that you might have had a negative experience while trying to get help for your pain, from structural issues (the brevity of visits with your practitioner) to temporary solutions (pain meds dispensed from the emergency room). It is important to understand that pain assessment is difficult, especially for chronic pain. There are no good tests. Most pain improves after a short period of time, and because drugs have side effects, most practitioners want to wait and see. But that doesn't mean you can't advocate for yourself and work with your practitioner to manage your pain.

Here are some questions to ask your practitioners about your pain:

What can I do to help prevent pain?
Are there supplements or lifestyle modifications you recommend for treating my pain?
If I get injured, what are the best ways I can take care of myself?

It is important to acknowledge that pain has a psychological (mental) component to it. Many practitioners will ask that you work on this part of your pain experience through therapy or other activities that do not involve medication. You owe it to yourself to try multiple methods of pain relief, including therapy.

How Can You Help Your Body Be Less Sensitive to Pain?

We often feel like we have to categorize our pain and make it make sense, but sometimes it won't make sense. It is not your fault if you can't distract your brain from your pain. If you have strong feelings of guilt, shame, and weakness, understand that these feelings are common with chronic pain and long illness. In no way are we suggesting that you can just "think your way" out of pain. But there are some cognitive tricks and things you can do to prepare yourself and maybe even to rewire your pain signals. Apps and workbooks, as well as pain psychologists and other pain professionals, can give you tools that help your body learn a different way to process pain by creating new neural pathways.

Learn about pain. The more you know about something and how it works, the less scary it is. There are several great apps and workbooks that can teach you more about pain. The more you know, the more likely you are to feel a sense of understanding, control, and peace and to feel your pain lessening.

Recognize what your pain is trying to tell you. What can you do to listen better and be a better partner with your pain? While there is rarely a magic eraser for pain, it can shift, and these tools can help you reduce pain as a barrier to living your life.

CHAPTER 5

Long Fatigue

I started having chronic fatigue right when I first got sick. It was this heaviness I had never experienced before. It didn't matter how much I slept, or if I ate regularly. I had lead pumping through my veins. Heavy and unmotivated. Like the exhausted feeling from the flu, except it never goes away.

Some tiredness improves with rest or a short break. But in a long illness, fatigue can be a constant. Eyelids begin to sag halfway through a magazine article. After a full night's sleep, you may be ready to go back to bed. Rest doesn't feel restful. People once full of vigor are now riddled with self-doubt. They feel deflated and confused. They can experience a profound and haunting loss of identity.

What You Will Learn in This Chapter:

- Causes of fatigue and the medical care you need
- Key information about myalgic encephalomyelitis/chronic fatigue syndrome (ME/CFS)
- Treatment options, including natural products and pacing exercise therapy
- Information about your mitochondria, the energy batteries of your body
- Evidence-based recovery tools, including CBT-inspired exercises, mindful movement, and activity logs

Investigating Fatigue

Fatigue can be a symptom of a number of illnesses, but it can also be the primary problem itself. There are many potential causes of fatigue, including:

Anxiety

Autoimmune disorders

Blood conditions

Cancer

Depression

Dysautonomia and autonomic dysfunction

Genetic mutations

Heart conditions

Hormone imbalance

Lung conditions

Menopause

Myalgic encephalomyelitis/chronic fatigue syndrome (ME/CFS)

Poor nutrition

Post-concussive syndrome

Post-infectious syndromes

Post-traumatic stress disorder

Rheumatologic disease

Sleep problems

Vitamin deficiencies

Your primary practitioner is a good starting point for ruling out obvious medical causes, like anemia or breathing problems. This workup often involves lab tests and a mental health screening, and sometimes a sleep study is suggested. Labs commonly look at the functioning of your blood cells, immune system, endocrine system, including different hormones, and digestive system.

When the medical workup is inconclusive, some people are diagnosed with ME/CFS. In our experience, it is always worthwhile to get a second opinion, as extreme fatigue may be masking another condition; for example, heart failure or sleep apnea may show up only as fatigue. It is a common misconception that you can't have ME/CFS and another condition, but you can. Getting an appropriate medical evaluation is essential.

We will highlight ME/CFS because it is a commonly diagnosed long illness, but this chapter is pertinent to *any* kind of fatigue. We will also give you tools to help you understand and work with your fatigue.

What Is ME/CFS?

Symptoms of ME/CFS include fatigue, worsening symptoms after exercise, unrefreshing sleep, brain fog, and dizziness. This diagnosis is given when symptoms persist past six months and there is no clear alternative medical explanation. What differentiates ME/CFS from other diagnoses is post-exertional fatigue: feeling more tired after exertion or exercise rather than refreshed or energized.

After receiving the diagnosis, our patients are often left with more questions than answers. Although we still don't know as much as we need to know about this condition, research has revealed the following:

There can be genetic roots and genetic differences in people with ME/CFS.

Infections can trigger ME/CFS.

In most cases of ME/CFS, the immune system isn't working optimally.

There are probably differences in mitochondria (the body's energy batteries) in people with ME/CFS and problems with detoxification pathways.

Autoimmunity—the body not recognizing parts of itself—is probably involved in many cases of ME/CFS.

Gut health issues are involved. You'll read more on this in Chapter 9, but in short, the gut microbiome of people with ME/CFS does not have as many microbe species and lacks enough healthy microbes.

Treatment for Fatigue

Exhaustion can feel like it will last forever. But fatigue can shift, lift, and change. There is no one-size-fits-all solution. We have therapies to help treat it, although there is no magic pill that works overnight. Our best evidence for successful treatment of chronic fatigue comes from cognitive behavioral therapy for people experiencing specific symptoms, mind-body therapies, and exercise. Later we also address pharmacological therapies. In our clinics, we focus on anti-inflammatory strategies and optimization of sleep and exercise. We stay up to date on the latest research and are constantly looking for more options for our patients.

Some practitioners offer treatments for people with fatigue and ME/CFS that have not been shown to improve the illness, have high costs, are not covered by insurance, and can have serious side effects. It is understandable that people would search for a cure. But be aware that there are practitioners who prey on this instinct and offer treatments that can be harmful.

The best way to protect yourself is to check with national support groups for your illness to see if the treatment you are interested in has been addressed in their guidelines and also to reach out to experts in the field. Never start a treatment without doing your homework and having multiple practitioners weighing in.

Cognitive Behavioral Therapy

Fatigue isn't just in your head, and it is invalidating to recommend psychological treatment alone. But fatigue is emotionally taxing and can generate emotional patterns that push against recovery, not toward it.

Many people find that their fatigue shifts only when they are also exploring the psychological ties to fatigue. Studies have shown that cognitive behavioral therapy (CBT) can lessen fatigue and improve mood, because it focuses on the connections between your thoughts, your feelings, and your body. CBT helps you see how fatigue is connected to your thinking and emotions. It is nearly impossible not to have fatigue impact your emotions. Relentless exhaustion changes the body and mind. The way we relate to fatigue can change the way we experience fatigue. CBT may or may not be a treatment you choose, but if you are feeling pulled toward understanding the psychological connections between fatigue and your emotional life, CBT may be a good place to start.

When we feel fatigued, we often feel anxious, scared, or (justifiably) angry. It makes sense that these feelings may be fueled by self-defeating and hopeless thoughts. Fatigue can sit like a heavy weight on your life, with devastating results. These emotional responses are human and understandable, but they may pull you into a pattern of avoidance. When you avoid things like moving your body or taking care of yourself, your fatigue will often get worse.

Take a moment to look at the triangle diagram here, showing how thoughts, feelings, and behaviors are connected in chronic fatigue. In this example, a person with fatigue thinks, "This will never get better." That thought brings up feelings of sadness and frustration. Then, rather than go for a walk, they decide to stay home. The more they avoid physical activity, the weaker they feel. That weakness causes more fatigue. The fatigue worsens the person's sadness, which leads them to avoid activity even more. This is how the mind gets into a cycle that works against healing. It's a feedback loop.

"This will never get better"
THOUGHTS

BEHAVIORS
Staying home instead of
going out for a walk

FEELINGS
Sad, angry, frustrated

Journaling

In CBT, the relationship between your thoughts, feelings, and behaviors are examined more fully. Take a moment to see if you can connect your feelings, thoughts, and behaviors to your experience with fatigue.

In your journal, create your own triangle and answer the following questions:

Thoughts: What thoughts come up when you think of fatigue?
Feelings: What feelings arise when you feel fatigued?
Behaviors: What behaviors do you engage in when thoughts and feelings about fatigue arise?

When you notice these thoughts, feelings, and behaviors as you go through your day, slow down. Once you are aware of them, you can get closer to understanding their relationship to your fatigue. Ideally, it is best to connect with a therapist with expertise working with fatigue. There are several CBT-for-fatigue workbooks listed in the resources section in the back of this book.

Mind-Body Therapies

In a haze of fatigue, you may neglect your body. Mind-body therapies can reconnect you to your body, unlocking any stagnation or tension contributing to your fatigue. Qigong and tai chi, Asian healing practices that combine movement with breathing, have been shown in studies to be potentially beneficial. Studies show that acupuncture is helpful for some people in reducing their fatigue. (See Chapter 20 on traditional medicine for more information.) Massage is also an evidence-based therapy recommended for fatigue, and it's readily available in most cities. Lower-cost massage can be accessed at massage training schools and through some massage membership programs. Your insurance or FSA may cover therapeutic massage as well.

Supplements and Natural Products

Many of our patients want to try a supplement to combat their fatigue. Regrettably, the medical evidence for the efficacy of many supplements for fatigue is not very strong. But there are two exceptions. If your vitamin D level is low, then starting a vitamin D supplement can improve your energy levels. This is also true for vitamin B_{12}. Your primary care practitioner can easily order both tests.

Although we cannot strongly recommend any supplement for fatigue, there are five supplements that we use judiciously in our patients with chronic fatigue, with some positive results: acetyl-L-carnitine, NADH (nicotinamide adenine dinucleotide), ginseng, turmeric, and coenzyme Q_{10}. Each of these has been studied in fatigue conditions and *may* have benefits.

If you are thinking about starting a supplement, always talk to your health care practitioner to make sure it is safe for you. When chosen incorrectly, supplements can interact with other medicines and even worsen certain health conditions. (See Chapter 21 on supplements and natural products.)

Medications

Treating fatigue with medication requires an accurate understanding of the cause. For example, fatigue from a thyroid condition should be treated with thyroid medication. Fatigue from a sleep disorder or depression might be addressed with a combination of medication and psychological treatments. But what about the fatigue that has no clear underlying cause other than long illness?

Currently, despite research, there is no medication with strong evidence behind it for treating fatigue directly. Psychotropic medications like antidepressants can be useful in people who have depression or high anxiety as well as fatigue. After a discussion of risks and benefits, your practitioner may also try a stimulant medication (like Ritalin or Adderall), but it is unclear how well these work over the long term. Some practitioners, including ourselves, are using low-dose naltrexone (see page 65) for chronic fatigue because of its effects on the immune system and its low-risk profile. But this medication is used off-label—which means that it is not always covered by insurance—and we still await further studies to help us assess its long-term viability.

Many other medications specifically for ME/CFS have been studied, including immunosuppressive medications like steroids and immuno-globulins. They have not shown sustained improvement in fatigue and have significant side effects. The same is true for treatment with antiviral medications.

Do You Need High-Dose Vitamins for Your Fatigue? Could a Mutation in the MTHFR Gene Be Responsible?

We order homocysteine testing for almost all of our patients with fatigue. Why? Because some people have dangerous mutations in the methylenetet-rahydrofolate reductase (MTHFR) gene that cause vitamin imbalances with potentially severe consequences, including increased risk of fatigue, head-ache, blood clots, depression, dementia, and heart disease. Once the diag-nosis is made and treatment is initiated, people finally start feeling better.

Testing for homocysteine is a cost-effective way to screen for one of these dangerous mutations and get a person with fatigue started right away on the correct treatment. Homocysteine is an amino acid that is a by-product of the breakdown of proteins. High levels of homocysteine can cause prob-lems in your body, ultimately damaging your arteries and veins. People who have certain long illnesses or who have low vitamin B_6, vitamin B_{12}, or folate levels can have high levels of homocysteine. Low levels of vitamins and ele-vated homocysteine can happen because of a mutation in the MTHFR gene. Mutations in this gene are very common: 40 to 60 percent of the population have at least one mutated gene, and 25 to 30 percent have a mutation in both genes. Dangerous mutations in the MTHFR gene prevent your body from turning vitamin B_{12}, vitamin B_6, and folate into forms it can use. These vitamins are vital to body functioning. For example, folate is essential in making *neurotransmitters*, the chemicals that regulate your mood.

There is strong evidence that significant harm is caused by only certain mutations in both copies of your MTHFR genes (although we find that even one mutation can impact long illness). Since genetic testing is expensive and hard to access, we recommend starting with a test of your homocysteine level to understand your risk. People who have the MTHFR mutation but also normal homocysteine levels do not regularly need vitamin supplementation.

If you have low vitamin levels and a high homocysteine level, treatment with high-dose vitamins to correct these imbalances can be transformative. This simple test is worth discussing with your primary practitioner, especially if you have ever had a history of low B_{12}, low folate, or other vitamin deficiencies.

Sleep

Getting restful sleep is essential to any treatment plan for ME/CFS and general fatigue. Of course, despite being exhausted, many of our patients still feel unrefreshed by sleep, or they have difficulty with nighttime sleep. If you have insomnia along with fatigue, treating the insomnia is a good place to start. Studies show that treating insomnia reduces daytime fatigue. There are also sleep disorders that cause you to feel unusually tired during the day and to fall asleep frequently, even when you don't want to. Learn more about insomnia and drowsiness in Chapter 10.

Exercise

Exercise is essential to decrease your fatigue. Without movement, it is unlikely that you will feel better. Even in its smallest doses of one to two minutes at a time of walking or lifting your limbs in bed, exercise releases chemicals that promote a decreased sense of fatigue, making it easier to do simple tasks. Inactivity causes your muscles to break down. Hundreds of studies have shown that fatigue improves with exercise.

The general recommendation for adults is to perform 150 minutes of *aerobic exercise* weekly—that is, running, walking, and similar exercises that get you out of breath—plus two or three sessions of strength training. That can be too much for someone with fatigue. The trick is to get in small amounts of exercise and then build up slowly to the recommended exercise dose. Luckily, as little as one- or two-minute increments of how much you exercise can improve your health.

This effect has even been proven in those with ME/CFS. *Pacing exercise therapy* involves starting exercise with small increments, going slow, and gradually increasing how much you exercise so you don't overdo it. For all people with extreme fatigue, it is essential to work with health care practitioners to connect you to coaches, trainers, and therapists who will come up with a movement plan that is right for you. Just remember to take it slow when you start out. (For more on exercise, see Chapter 19.)

What Is Post-Exertional Malaise or Fatigue? Do You Have It? Will It Keep You from Exercising?

When people exercise, they feel better afterward. If they exercise hard, they might also notice soreness and a need for a little more sleep. What people who have ME/CFS experience after pushing themselves too hard is very different. Post-exertional malaise following a physical or cognitive activity can last for hours, days, or weeks and result in an exacerbation, or flare, of ME/CFS symptoms.

A flare can be triggered by something as simple as going on a walk or going sofa shopping. These flares are not relieved by taking a bath and taking it easy for a few days. They can last for weeks or months, greatly limiting a person's ability to take care of themselves. And some flares don't resolve. During a flare from post-exertional malaise, symptoms such as cognitive dysfunction (like brain fog) and orthostatic intolerance (such as dizziness) greatly increase, and other symptoms might return as well. Talk with your practitioners if you are concerned that post-exertional malaise might be an issue for you.

Here is a story from one person with ME/CFS about navigating exercise:

I'd always been really into exercise. I ran a marathon, I built my own house, I worked in search and rescue and could hike long distances. I took a lot of pleasure in exercise. Then the fatigue started. It felt like I couldn't downshift to get more power like I used to—I had to drag myself up a hill. If I exercised too much, I felt terrible the next day. I could feel lousy for weeks.

Eventually I was diagnosed with CFS. At that time doctors didn't even address the issue of exercise, even though it was an important part of my life and it's such a key issue for managing ME/CFS.

Through experimentation, I realized that the absolute key to achieving any kind of functionality was being really careful when exerting myself. I had to pay close attention to my body to detect early signals of getting tired, and to stop. Not in five minutes, but immediately. Once I learned to recognize and listen to those very early signals of fatigue, my flares became less frequent.

The amazing thing now is that exercise makes me feel better. I deal with a lot of back pain. And if I go swimming, my back pain goes away, and it stays away the rest of the day. So I'm really motivated. My experience of exercise making me sick was scary, but the idea that CFS patients are afraid of exercise is the wrong way for doctors to think. As soon as my body was capable, the first thing I wanted to do was exercise and see what I could do.

Nutrition

Along with exercise, we recommend an anti-inflammatory diet to combat ME/CFS and general fatigue. Since immune system dysregulation appears to be a factor in the development of this disease, reducing inflammation through diet is a part of most treatment plans. (See Chapter 18 to learn more.)

Gut Health

We discuss gut health in detail in Chapter 9, but it's worth mentioning here. Since the gut microbiome in people with ME/CFS is often out of balance, researchers are looking at the role of treatments targeting gut bacteria. We think it's important to understand the role of your microbiome in your overall health, especially if you are fatigued.

Mitochondria and Energy Levels

Exhaustion and fatigue are near-universal features of long illness. To understand why, we start at the cellular level. Your body's energy storage and production systems hold the key to your body's ability to produce energy, fight fatigue, and protect your body from inflammation.

Energy metabolism is the process by which your body converts the food, water, and oxygen you consume into energy. Proteins are broken down into amino acids (the most basic components of proteins), fats into fatty acids, and carbohydrates into sugars. Once these simple products get into your cells, they are taken apart by a complex set of reactions to power your body. Excess energy is stored in special fat cells called adipocytes. Accessing stored energy requires coordinated hormone signals. As with any complex procedure, energy metabolism is susceptible to mistakes along the way.

Energy is generated in the factories of your cells, the mitochondria. Every cell in your body (except red blood cells) has hundreds of them. They have their own genes, called mitochondrial DNA (mtDNA), because long ago they were their own organism before they joined your cells. Mitochondria were so awesome at converting oxygen into energy that other organisms absorbed them and they became part of us. Your mitochondria are essentially batteries for your body. The air you breathe and the food you eat charge that battery.

All the mitochondria in a cell are in contact, communicating with each other about what is going on in their part of the cell. They sense fluctuations in stress and sex hormones, blood pressure, and even how much ice cream you just ate. They know when you are sleeping, they know when you're awake. They are completely in tune with your body.

Since the mitochondria know all the gossip, they influence the activity of the cell and get it to send signals to your body. If things are quiet, they may lie low and relax. If things are busy or stressful, they ramp up. Sometimes the stress for the mitochondria is too much and they get damaged. And the body treats damaged mitochondria as a foreign invader.

WHAT MAKES THE MITOCHONDRIA

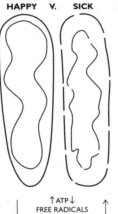

HAPPY   V.   SICK

• ANTI–INFLAMMATORY
• PLANT–BASED DIET
• HIGH IN ANTIOXIDANTS,
FIBER, MINERALS, AND VITAMINS
• INTUITIVE EATING
• ADEQUATE HYDRATION
• REGULAR EXERCISE
• RESTFUL SLEEP
• OPTIMIZED BREATHING
• MICROBIOME DIVERSITY
• MANAGED STRESS
• GENETICS

• ULTRA–PROCESSED DIET
LOW IN FIBER; HIGH IN
SUGAR, BAD FATS, AND MEAT
• ROUTINE OVERCONSUMPTION
• <1.5 L WATER DAILY
• EXTREME OR MINIMAL
EXERCISE
• POOR SLEEP QUALITY AND
QUANTITY
• POOR OXYGENATION
• LIMITED MICROBIOME
• HIGH STRESS
• POLLUTION AND TOXINS
• UV RADIATION ☼
• SMOKING
• ALCOHOL AND DRUGS
• MEDICATION
• GENETICS
• AGING

↑ATP↓
FREE RADICALS
OXIDATIVE STRESS
INFLAMMATION
↓ DISEASE PROGRESSION

How Do Your Daily Activities Affect Your Mitochondria?

Supporting your mitochondria can be thought of as charging your batteries. Fatigue is the result when that battery runs low. One reason that happens is that mitochondria can't keep up with the behaviors and choices of an average Western lifestyle. Low physical activity, ultra-processed foods, bad breathing habits, poor sleep, and high stress cause life-altering changes in cell metabolism. In response to all of this cellular stress, your cells make more mitochondria. Quickly made mitochondria are sometimes damaged and can't run smoothly, causing the body's battery to run dangerously low. It is useful to explore what supports your mitochondria and to make small shifts toward supporting their health.

Journaling

WHAT MAKES YOUR MITOCHONDRIA HAPPY?

Think of a time when you felt like you had a lot of energy and fatigue wasn't a big issue. This was probably a time when your mitochondria were happy. Describe this time in your journal.

Example: Happy = going on a walk, laughing with friends, eating a diet with less sugar.

Now think of a time when you felt like you had low energy or fatigue. This might have been a time when your mitochondria were overwhelmed.

Example: Sick = eating lots of fast food, staying inside on the couch all day, obsessing about work/project.

Look at what you wrote in the "happy" column versus the "sick" column. What are things you wrote in the happy column that you can do more of? What are things you wrote in the sick column that you feel like you can change? Are there things you cannot change? Circle the things you think you could make small changes to and draw Xs next to those you don't think you can change now. In a few weeks or months, come back to this page in your journal. You might be surprised to see that you're ready to turn some of those Xs into circles.

There are many causes of fatigue. It is tempting to imagine that you have a single treatable cause of your fatigue, but for many people that is not the case. Although a silver-bullet cure for fatigue isn't available, there are tools and lifestyle changes that can improve the symptoms.

With the help of your team, start to add the tools in this chapter to your routine and find a combination that works for you.

EXERCISE

MINDFULNESS: BODY SCANNING WITH MOVEMENT

MRI studies of the brain show that *thinking* about exercising can be as powerful as *actually* exercising. Many professional athletes use these techniques to practice while they are resting or injured. Let's get your brain moving!

Find a safe space to lie down. A comfortable chair can also work. Consider having someone else read this to you or record yourself reading this and play it back.

Brief instruction: Starting at your toes and going up to your head, focus on a part of your body and then move that part of your body. At the end, shake your whole body. Then be still and breathe deeply. It's okay if your ability to move is limited. Just move your body in any way that feels right for you.

In-depth explanation:

Take three slow, deep breaths. Imagine that everything in your room is melting away and you see just yourself, floating on the floor. You are safe and strong. Continue slow, deep breathing throughout this exercise.

Bring your awareness to your body. Bring your attention to your toes and feet. Gently move your feet in different ways: wiggle and spread your toes, flex and point your feet, roll your ankles in a circle. If you have limited movement in a part of your body, respect your own limits, and move in any way that feels right for you.

Scan up through the rest of your body: legs, arms, pelvis, belly, neck, and head. At each area, focus on maintaining your deep breathing while allowing your body to gently explore movement.

At each area of your body, remember what that part of your body can do when you feel strong. Imagine kicking a ball, picking up a box, carrying groceries, dancing, hugging someone.

Now move your entire body in whatever way is comfortable for you. This might mean shaking and wiggling out your head, arms, and legs, all moving together, awake and ready to start the day. Your body is full of the memories of being strong in the past. You are full of peace and knowledge that you will soon move that way again.

Come to a still position and take three deep breaths, in and out. Slowly open your eyes.

Journaling

Think about the following questions and record your thoughts in your journal:

What tools do I have to address my fatigue? Are there any new strategies I want to try?

The most important thing I learned is that even if I do all the things to prevent fatigue, like drinking water, eating consistently, exercising, sleeping, there are just going to be times when that is not enough. And I will just be exhausted sometimes. I've found that giving myself grace and pacing myself, I learned to acknowledge that I was fatigued, to sit down and take a break until I feel a little better, and get up again. What I can and can't do is different, and that is okay.

EXERCISE

ACTIVITY LOG

We've talked about movement and exercise being great antidotes to fatigue, but any and all activity can help too. Sometimes we aren't even aware of how active we are during our day. This log is designed to help you understand your current activity level by looking at a whole week, or even a month. Once you know where you are, you can set realistic goals. Each day write down all of your activities in which you were moving your body. We have included examples to help you identify when you are being active.

At the top of a page in your journal, write down a goal. At the end of each day, list what you did that day and for how long. At the end of the week, review the log without judgment. You are healing from an illness with significant fatigue. At the start, you may have engaged in almost no activity. That's okay.

For the next week, write down a new goal at the top of a page. Tailor the goal to your body today, not to what you "should" be doing. If you have trouble coming up with activity goals, try reviewing the examples here.

Examples of Activity

> *Low difficulty: Standing, short walks, housework (dishes), preparing food, restorative yoga (YouTube or virtual class)* (Note: *Most of our patients choose items from the low-difficulty category initially and slowly build up to moderate activity.*)

Moderate difficulty: Chair yoga, physical therapy exercises, housework (weeding, mopping), long walks, tai chi

High difficulty: Yoga or Pilates class, jogging/running, strength training, hiking

Examples of Goals

Keep an activity log

Walk ten minutes longer each day

Exercise for ten more minutes each day

Take five laps around the house

Do physical therapy three times per week

Do five minutes of standing housework each day

SAMPLE LOG

Goal: Keep an activity log

Date	Activity	Thoughts
Sunday	Did housework for fifteen minutes in the morning Made a big pot of soup for lunches this week	
Monday	PT exercises before work for fifteen minutes Thirty-minute slow walk after dinner	
Tuesday	Raked leaves from the front lawn for twenty minutes	
Wednesday	Used standing desk at work for fifteen minutes each hour	
Thursday	PT exercises before work for fifteen minutes	
Friday	Raining outside, so I did a thirty-minute yoga video	
Saturday	Took a hike in the park for an hour	

CHAPTER 6

Breathing and Lung Concerns

*When my disease is flaring, I have to take the elevator instead of the stairs.
I love exercise, so it makes me mad when I am having problems with feeling
short of breath. I am embarrassed because I seem out of shape. I get anxious
because I feel like I can't breathe. Which makes everything worse. It makes
other people around me anxious. Once I learned more about how your brain
and lungs are connected, it motivated me to do breathing exercises. I have
become much more comfortable with being breathless, and I feel like my body
knows more of what to do now to calm myself down.*

What You Will Learn in This Chapter:

- The critical role of your lungs in your overall health
- Ways to investigate underlying lung problems
- How to use the brain-lung connection to help with your breathing
- Exercises to strengthen your breathing

Many people with a long illness suffer from shortness of breath. It can
feel like not enough air is getting in, and you are already gasping for
the next breath. Or it may just feel like your breathing is never easy. You
may experience difficult breathing while resting, or only with exercise.

If you have this problem and have not spoken with your practitioner yet,
start with questions like these:

It feels like I can never get enough air in. Why is this?

Have I had all of the tests I need to make sure there isn't something else
going on?

What do my tests show?

Is pulmonary rehabilitation right for me?

What exercises can I do to improve my breathing?

If it's still not clear after your practitioner responds, it's okay to ask for more information:

Can you draw a picture showing what is happening in my lungs?

Can you try to use less medical language?

Can you show me how to do the breathing exercises while I am in your office?

This chapter will give you a foundation for lung health. We introduce exercises to help strengthen your breathing. With knowledge and skills, you can better understand the path to recovery from shortness of breath. The lungs are complex, so let's start by demystifying breathing.

Breathing 101

You breathe 20,000 times per day. Breathing plays a critical role in many functions of the body: blood pressure, mood, cognition, digestion, athletic performance, and immunity.

Many of us just don't think about breathing, which is natural and unconscious—until it is not. Your lungs are surrounded by 10 pounds of muscles. Each muscle plays a role in the delicate dance of breathing, and even the slightest change can make the process more or less efficient.

Your lungs contain 1,500 miles of airways and 250 million to 500 million alveoli to accomplish vital functions. They also depend on the chest muscles, heart, blood vessels, and nervous system to work properly. Damage to any part of the respiratory system, not just the lungs themselves, can lead to problems breathing.

Lung Function Tests

Lung function tests, also called pulmonary function tests (PFTs), are ordered by your pulmonologist (lung specialist) or primary care practitioner for most lung conditions. This series of tests is called *spirometry*. Spirometry measures your lung capacity—the amount of air the lungs can hold—and how forcefully and quickly you can empty the air. It also compares the amount of air that escapes your lungs with how much total air is in your lungs.

These simple tests provide answers to the following questions:

Are you getting all of the air out of your lungs, or is some air getting trapped?
Are you getting enough air into your lungs?
Are your lungs expanding enough?

Sometimes medication is given during these tests to see if your lung function changes in response, such as in testing for asthma. Other tests that help practitioners understand complementary aspects of lung function, develop treatment plans, and decide what other specialists might be helpful include the following:

Lung volume test
Diffusion capacity test, which measures how well oxygen gets into your blood
Exercise testing, which looks at what happens to your breathing with
     exercise and how your heart is working during exercise
Testing the strength of the muscles of breathing

If your lung function tests are abnormal, these tests are often repeated over time to gain information about how your disease or treatment is progressing. Your practitioner might also order other tests to help investigate specific abnormalities or check for other related conditions:

Blood tests
Pulse oxygen saturation (a small device attached to your finger or ear)

Imaging (X-rays, CT scans, MRI)

Testing of heart function

We have a lot of tests to help with establishing a diagnosis. But sometimes the results of all of these tests are normal even if you have shortness of breath.

When the Tests Don't Explain What's Wrong

Often we find an abnormality from our testing, but I warn my patients that this might not explain everything that they are feeling. Lung function and other types of tests help us to make sure a potentially life-threatening condition is not causing the problem. We are making sure that it is safe for them to engage in physical activity, which is what will help the body heal after all injury and illness. Even when the testing points to a specific condition that may be causing shortness of breath, there is still a process of trial and error. In clinic, we continue to work with patients to make lifestyle changes and trial medications to see what helps them specifically, as each person is different.

—Brendan Huang, MD, PhD, pulmonologist at the
University of California–San Francisco

Many people with shortness of breath feel disheartened when the tests don't reflect their suffering, as has happened with many people who have long Covid. If that is your situation, your practitioner probably has made sure to test you for other conditions that can masquerade as lung problems, including heart problems, blood pH problems, and anemia.

If all tests are normal, the process can be frustrating. But keep in mind that your lung problem can still be improved. Let's explore how lungs heal, and what can be done to optimize breathing.

Lung Injury and Healing

After most short infections of the lungs, there is short-term (*acute*) inflammation, which resolves. But we know that some inflammation doesn't go away. If it is bad enough in the lungs, inflammation can cause thickening and stiffening of the lungs, called *fibrosis*. When fibrosis has developed, the damage is usually not reversible. This doesn't mean that you can't improve your breathing to some degree, only that the affected areas of your lungs are not likely to regenerate. If you are worried about fibrosis, ask your practitioner to review your diagnosis with you. Fibrosis can be seen on CT scans and some other imaging.

A large proportion of lung dysfunction, especially immediately after illness, is caused by a phenomenon called *atelectasis*. Portions of the lungs collapse on themselves, preventing oxygen absorption, and the body doesn't get the optimal amount of nutrients, resulting in shortness of breath. Atelectasis primarily is caused by *immobility and deconditioning* (the medical term for the loss of strength that happens from a lack of activity). When you are less active, the muscles that support your breathing also get weaker. The less you move, the harder breathing will be.

There is good and bad news: you can get better, but the treatment is physical activity. We recognize that the advice to increase how much you exercise when you are short of breath can be frustrating to hear. But it really is the best way to strengthen your breathing. Exercise not only opens the lungs but helps them to stay clean and to heal. Physical activity helps to clear out both mucus and debris. It also strengthens the muscles that support your breathing. Remember to discuss starting exercise with your practitioner, who may have helpful tips or can make a referral to physical therapy. Skip to Chapter 19 to learn more about gently introducing more activity into your life in a way that feels right for you.

Other lifestyle changes that can improve your lung hygiene include improving your posture—keeping your chest straight and wide open to maximize the amount of space available for air movement and to strengthen your core muscles. For people with neck and back problems, it can be beneficial to work with a physical therapist specifically around posture. This work can strengthen weak muscles and slowly unwind tight muscles, which compromise your ability to get full, deep breaths. Immediately after illness, using certain simple pieces of equipment, such as an incentive spirometer (a handheld device you take breaths in), can also ensure that you are maximizing your recovery by taking large breaths throughout the day.

The Lung-Brain Connection

Examining the relationship between your emotions and your breathing can be vitally important to optimizing your pulmonary recovery. Your brain communicates to your lungs, and vice versa. Your brain also changes the rate of your breathing and can coordinate how fast you breathe to match your activity levels. More recently, a direct connection found between the *amygdala*, your brain's fear control center, and the lungs shows that your breathing is tied to your fear response. We also know that increased stress hormone levels can delay pulmonary healing.

It is also easy to fall into a pattern in which fear and anxiety from difficulty breathing worsen your anxiety. It's a vicious cycle. For example, when the person in this diagram starts to exercise, fear and anxiety around developing shortness of breath arise. Those feelings are connected to negative thoughts, and together, the feelings, negative thoughts, and body sensations lead the person to stop exercising.

It is nearly impossible to experience shortness of breath without developing some amount of fear or anxiety, some of which is probably unavoidable.

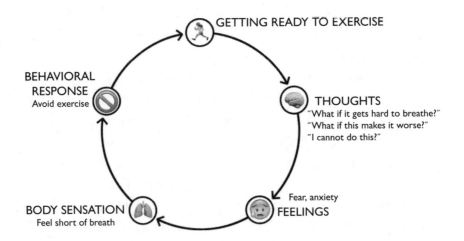

GETTING READY TO EXERCISE

BEHAVIORAL
RESPONSE
Avoid exercise

THOUGHTS
"What if it gets hard to breathe?"
"What if this makes it worse?"
"I cannot do this?"

BODY SENSATION
Feel short of breath

Fear, anxiety
FEELINGS

Your fear and anxiety can be alleviated to some extent when test results are normal or when objective tests help you come to a better understanding of your lung function. You can also use CBT skills (see Chapter 10) to try to understand why you experience shortness of breath with exercise.

You can disrupt this pattern by recognizing when you are pouring gasoline on the fire. Sometimes the fear of shortness of breath begins before you even have trouble breathing. This fearful anticipation of the sensation of difficulty breathing can actually bring it on. Similarly, distressing thoughts connected to your breathing can crank up your anxiety, which programs the brain to avoid things connected to difficult breathing, like movement or breathing exercises. On the superhighway of the mind, thoughts, feelings, body sensations, and behaviors all interconnect.

Having awareness of your own patterns around breathing is the first step to improving it.

Journaling

Re-create your personal version of this cycle.

What is the situation?
What are your feelings?
What are your body sensations?
What are your thoughts?
What are your behaviors?
What thoughts and emotions are connected to your breathing?

Pulmonary rehab was pretty helpful. But it's also just doing exercises to build up that stamina. You don't realize how important posture is to breathing. Even making sure that you have some level of fitness. If you are unable to get out of bed at the time, just trying to make sure you're sitting up every day or trying to get to the chair, working to change the position of your body against gravity.

A couple of other things that I found really helpful. One was being able to get back into swimming. I think that controlled rhythmic breathing was really helpful to reduce that sensation of shortness of breath. Yoga is another option where you're doing a lot of controlled breathing and a lot of rhythmic breathing. I also found singing helpful since it focused on breath control and stamina. Even little things like blowing bubbles (from soap or in the bathtub), blowing paper across a table with a straw—it may seem silly, but it can be a big help towards getting better breathing.

Improve Your Breathing...with Breathing

Evidence has shown that breathing exercises can improve quality of life, decrease shortness of breath, strengthen breathing muscles, lessen anxiety and depression, and increase exercise capacity.

Breathing also regulates the nervous system. When we are anxious, we hold our breath. Anxiety is a fight-or-flight response in the sympathetic nervous system. Why would we need to breathe deeply if we're running from a tiger? So preexisting anxiety can worsen the experience of shortness of breath. Deep breaths strengthen the rest-and-digest parasympathetic nervous system. Most of our patients have an imbalance between the two parts of the nervous system. When you combine psychological work with breathing exercises, you address both sides of this system.

Breathing also trains the muscles that support your chest. The stronger these muscles are, the more supported your breath will be. Think of breathing exercises as a gym workout for these muscles. We have included some exercises here to get you started. In addition, a pulmonary therapist could develop a customized breath-strengthening plan for you.

One note before we begin: you might feel scared to try these exercises. Just take it slow and remember that you can always stop and regulate your breathing. As with everything else in this book, these exercises are intended to serve you. If you are concerned that they might not be right for you, try them with your practitioner first to be sure.

EXERCISE

ALTERNATE NOSTRIL BREATHING

You will use your thumbs to alternately cover your nostrils, and then you will alternate inhales and exhales between your left and right nostrils.

Take your right thumb and cover your right nostril while you inhale through the left nostril.

Cover the left nostril with your left thumb and exhale through your right nostril.

Take your next inhalation through your left nostril.

Alternate inhales and exhales through your left and right nostrils.

If you find that you need to blow your nose, go ahead and do so. Resume the exercise when you are done. We recommend setting a timer for two minutes and building stamina from there up to five minutes.

EXERCISE

4-7-8 BREATHING

In this exercise, you breathe in and out while counting in your head. The exact numbers do not matter very much. What matters more is breathing in slowly, holding the breath, and exhaling slowly. You can pick the numbers that work for you.

Inhale through your nose and do a mental count to four.

Hold your breath for a mental count to seven.

Exhale completely through your mouth, doing a mental count to eight.

Practice for four to six rounds.

EXERCISE

GUIDED IMAGERY: "BODY FILLED WITH BREATH"

Find a space where it feels safe to lie down, to sit comfortably, or to settle in whatever position best suits your body.

Gently close your eyes and simply notice your breathing.

*Notice any thoughts or feelings that arise in connection to your breathing.
If you can, allow these thoughts and feelings to travel out of your mind
on each exhale.*

Feel the air entering your nose. Feel your chest rise with the breath.

*Allow your body to expand in any way that feels comfortable to allow for
just a little more breath.*

*Each breath is bringing oxygen into your body. On your next inhale, envision
each cell in your body being nourished...just by breathing.*

*With the next inhale, feel oxygen reaching your brain...chest...arms...
abdomen...pelvis...arms...legs...fingers...and toes.*

Experience your breath...it is doing an important job.

*Continue deep breathing, extending your inhale and exhale to whatever
point feels comfortable for you. If your mind wanders, bring it back to
the breath, to the oxygen reaching your cells. Allow for small moments
of appreciation for the marvel that is...breath.*

CHAPTER 7

Headaches

Right around the time of my lupus diagnosis was when I started having migraines. I progressed to the point where I was having them daily. Headaches can be really isolating because some people don't get exactly what it's like. Some people think that headaches are willful. Oh God, the number of times I was told, "Well, have you drunk enough water today?" You know, they turn it into something that is your fault. And I'm like, trust me, if drinking water would make this stop, I would literally just sit on the toilet and have it go in one end and out the other.

And it's the same story as chronic illness, which becomes your fault, as opposed to the fault of some bad neurological connections in your brain.

What You Will Learn in This Chapter:

- Types of headaches in long illness and when to seek immediate medical attention
- Common migraine features and the neuroscience behind their intensity
- Treatments, from natural products to Botox injections
- Powerful lifestyle changes to reduce headaches
- Trigger management, self-massage, and other tools

What a Headache!

We use this saying to describe distressing, annoying, or uncomfortable experiences. For good reason. Headaches are painful and can be joined by other unpleasant symptoms: nausea, light sensitivity, fatigue, and brain fog (to name a few). They can be a response to many things, like stress, emotional fatigue, illness, and inflammation. The most common headaches in people with long illness are tension ("stress") headaches and migraine headaches. Tension headaches, which arise when you have higher levels of stress, you're dehydrated, or you've slept poorly, are generally mild and resolve with lifestyle changes. Migraines often do not.

The lifestyle changes we recommend for migraine headaches treat tension headaches as well. By focusing on migraines, we can address treatment for both headache types.

What Is a Migraine?

During a migraine, you can experience many different sensations in your body. These headaches hijack many territories of the brain by using the interconnected "superhighway" nervous system.

Your migraines will feel different depending upon the roads, or pathways, they take. We have included a checklist with the explanations here so that you can personalize the information you read. If you find yourself checking many boxes, this list can be helpful for talking to your health care practitioners.

Migraine Markers

Even if you have never had a headache, if you have a long illness you may be at increased risk for a migraine. Go through this checklist to see if you have any markers that increase your risk of migraine headaches:

Have You Experienced Any of These Migraine Markers?
Hangovers
Car sickness
Brain freeze (headaches with cold foods or drinks, like ice cream)
Colic as a baby
Frequent abdominal pain in childhood

Migraine Triggers

Many people can identify a reason why their headache started. This is a list of the common triggers for migraines. Once the trigger is pulled, the headache often follows.

Do Any of the Following Cause You to Have a Headache?
Skipping meals
Alcohol (especially wine)
Hangovers
Strong smells
Lights or sounds
Poor sleep
Weather
Dehydration
Hormone changes (often periods or menopause)

Do you have other headache triggers? List them in your journal.

Migraine Features

Migraines are rarely just a headache. A migraine spreads like a wave in the brain in a phenomenon called *cortical spreading depression*. This means that once the migraine begins, it has a domino effect. It spreads to parts of the brain that control other symptoms, like nausea, thinking, and vision.

Go through the list below to identify your headache features.

Do You Experience Any of the Following When You Have a Headache?
Pounding/pulsating pain
Neck pain
Nausea/vomiting
Vision changes/aura (shimmering or shapes in your vision)
Speech difficulties
Brain fog

Tingling
Feeling off-balance
Poor concentration
Dizziness
Light sensitivity
Sound sensitivity
Worsening with movement

We have listed only the most common features, but there are others. Do you have other symptoms in your body when you have headaches? Jot them down in your journal.

After Migraines

Migraines can hit you like a ton of bricks. It is common to experience changes even after the migraine has ended because your brain and body take time to recover from the stress of a migraine.

After Headaches, Do You Experience Any of the Following?
Hungover feeling
Exhaustion
Appetite changes (increased hunger or very little appetite)
Urinating more

I have a great PCP and neurologist, and with their help we have found that I have three different types of headaches. Each of them feels different and responds to a different treatment. Before working with them and using headache journals and reflecting on the headaches, I thought I was just having one type of headache that would respond to the treatment some of the time.

When Do You Need to Talk to a Medical Practitioner About Your Headaches?

If you are having any of the following symptoms, tell your health care team as soon as possible:

Headaches that are getting worse

Headaches that are stopping you from participating in daily activities,
   like your hobbies, your job, or family care

Headaches with fevers or chills

Headaches with bad neck pain and stiffness

Headaches and recent unintentional weight loss

New types of headaches

Headaches that get much worse when lying down

Headaches that get worse with exercise, lifting heavy things, coughing,
   or sexual activity

Headaches that started after a head injury

In rare instances, a headache is a sign of something more serious, like
bleeding in the brain. The following is a list of these serious signs. *If you have
a headache with any of these features, call 911 or go to the emergency department
right away:*

A headache that hits you suddenly and all at once, like a bolt of
   lightning

A headache that is *not* like your other headaches

A headache that is the worst one of your life

Neurologic symptoms that start suddenly (not slowly), like numbness,
   weakness, slurred speech, confusion, vertigo (room spinning), or
   vision loss, possibly indicating a stroke

When Headaches Start Somewhere Else

Some headaches start from other places in your body. It is common to see
headaches from problems in teeth, the jaw, or the sinuses. Treatment of
these headaches often requires seeing a dentist or ear, nose, and throat specialist (ENT).

Similarly, *cervicogenic headaches* originate from the cervical spine, which is in your neck. People with these headaches often need physical therapy and treatment of their spine problems before their headaches can get better.

What Is the Best Treatment for Headaches?

Your primary care practitioner can treat most headaches and will give you helpful guidance on lifestyle changes, medications, and referrals to physical therapy, which can be helpful for all types of headaches.

> I'm on one of the injectable migraine medications, and sometimes I'll go months without getting a migraine. It was just the most joyous moment when I realized I had gone months without having to stop my life to have a migraine.

If you are still suffering after following the advice of your primary care practitioner, ask for a referral to a neurologist. If your headaches aren't getting better with a neurologist managing them, ask for a referral to a headache specialist. These specialty neurologists focus on treating headaches and have many more tools for treating them. Headaches, especially migraines, are worth treating aggressively.

Many people also find relief with practitioners of integrative or alternative medicine. There are many ways to treat headaches. Here are examples of the ways in which we can treat migraine headaches.

Start with...	Talk to Your Primary Care Practitioner or Neurologist About...	Talk to a Headache Specialist About...
Lifestyle changes: Optimize exercise, improve diet, increase hydration, and increase restful sleep.	**"Abortive" medications:** Mostly anti-inflammatory pain medications or medications that target the spread of headache, these medicines stop a headache or prevent it from getting worse.	**Procedures:** Nerve block and Botox injections can both be effective in controlling migraines.

Headaches and food: Try cutting out the two best-known dietary headache triggers: alcohol (wine being the most common trigger) and nitrates or nitrites (the chemicals found primarily in cured meats like salami). Try to identify foods you ate when headache symptoms occurred. Chapters 17 and 18 on diet can help you further explore food journaling and elimination diets.	**"Preventive" medications:** These daily medicines work either on blood pressure or by adjusting chemical levels in the brain.	**Devices:** Electric or magnetic stimulation of the brain through medical devices can improve migraines.
Managing triggers: Use a headache diary to identify triggers and strategize ways to avoid them.	**Mind and body therapies:** Explore physical therapy, acupuncture, chiropractic care, massage, biofeedback, yoga, or mindfulness practice.	**Antibody therapy:** Antibody medications target inflammation levels in the brain.
	Natural products: Riboflavin (vitamin B_2) and magnesium are the most commonly used supplements to treat headaches. Many people also use melatonin when they have issues with both headaches and sleep. Melatonin can be used even without sleep problems to reduce migraines. Other supplements that have shown evidence for success in treating migraines include caffeine (usually in coffee or tea), coenzyme Q_{10}, curcumin, and ginger.	**Hospital-based treatment:** Some hospitals offer migraine treatments that involve intravenous infusions.

Journaling

When you get a headache, what do you usually do? What helps? What makes it worse?

After reading this chapter, did you learn anything that you want to talk to your health care practitioners about?

Trigger Management (aka Don't Pull the Trigger!)

If I have a glass of wine, I can guarantee that I will get a migraine. This is also true during periods of high stress and poor sleep. Knowing my triggers helps me have fewer headaches.

When we know our headache triggers, we can adjust our lifestyle to avoid them or reduce our exposure to them. Some triggers are easier to avoid than others. Once you identify a food in your diet as a trigger, you can be careful to avoid that food. Other triggers, however, are harder to avoid. A rainy day or cold temperatures may still cause a migraine, even if you bundle up and stay indoors.

Look at this list, note the triggers that apply to you, and write them in your journal.

Alcohol	Hormonal changes	Sounds
Certain foods	Lights	Stress
Dehydration	Poor sleep	Strong smells
Hangovers	Skipping meals	Weather

Now try writing out a plan to avoid these triggers where possible. Here are some examples:

Trigger: Hormone Changes

How will I manage this trigger?

    Talk to doc about options for managing my periods; rest more around the time of my period

Trigger: Poor Sleep

How will I manage this trigger?

    Read Chapter 10 on sleep and complete the exercises

    Take a class in CBT for insomnia

    Put down the phone an hour before bed

    Increase sunlight exposure during the day

HEADACHE DIARY

Most people don't remember all the details of their headaches when they're speaking with their practitioner. Keeping a headache diary, at least for a few months while you are figuring out the right treatment, can help you track your progress and understand trends in your headaches to unlock the best treatment.

You can re-create this sample diary in your journal or you can use the National Headache Foundation headache diary (which is available free on its website, headaches.org) to track your headaches this month. Bring your diary to your appointments so that your medical practitioners can understand your headaches better and develop the best plan for your treatment.

Date	Duration (Start and End Times)	Triggers	Severity (Worst Pain = 10; No Pain = 0)	Symptoms	Treatment Used	Relief (None, Some, Complete)
May 1	9:30 a.m.–11:00 a.m.	Poor sleep Glass of wine last night	7	Pounding pain Crankiness Craving for sugar beforehand Light/sound sensitivity Nausea Fatigue	Ibuprofen Caffeine (cup of coffee) Breathing exercise Cold pack on forehead Yoga stretches Rest	Some
May 1	6:00 p.m.–9:00 p.m.	Skipped lunch	5	Pounding pain Light sensitivity Nausea Fatigue	Ibuprofen Melatonin Yoga stretches Went to sleep	Complete
May 2	2:00 p.m.–4:00 p.m.	Started my period	7	Pounding pain Crankiness Light/sound sensitivity Nausea Fatigue (also the next day) Dizziness	Yoga stretches Cold pack on forehead Went to sleep	Some
May 3	8:00 a.m.–11:30 a.m.	Too much sun on a hike Dehydration	3	Pounding pain Nausea	Self-massage Drank water Rest (took a nap)	Complete

When Treating Headaches Causes Headaches

When headaches are bad enough, you may need a medication that ends the pain, like acetaminophen (Tylenol), ibuprofen (Advil or Motrin), or sumatriptan (or Imitrex), which are known as *abortive medications*. We think that taking pain-relieving medication too often changes how your brain understands pain and affects levels of inflammation.

Using too much abortive medication can bring on a *medication overuse headache*. In response, you need more medication to treat your headaches, gaining temporary relief but then a worsening headache.

If you are using pain medications most days for headaches, you may be trapped in this cycle. Talk to your practitioner about strategies to reduce your need for pain medications. This may mean taking a daily pill to prevent migraines or exploring other strategies for managing your pain.

EXERCISE

SELF-MASSAGE AND ACUPRESSURE

Self-massage is relaxing and can soften the muscles of the head and neck, which often tighten when a headache starts. This practice incorporates acupressure points inspired by traditional medicine.

We recommend starting self-massage when you do not have a headache. If it feels good to you, practice it daily for two weeks. Repeat the massage at the first sign of a headache. Use your headache diary to track your headaches and see if they reduce in frequency or intensity.

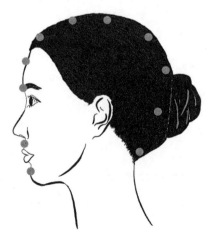

Midline Head Acupressure

> Start at the point at the base of your skull, where your head meets your neck. Using your second and third fingers, press firmly and apply continuous pressure. Slowly count to ten. Apply as much pressure as feels tolerable.

> Move to the next point, about three finger-breadths up, staying in the midline of your head. Press firmly and apply continuous pressure. Slowly count to ten.

> Continue to move up the back of your head and then down your face, pressing on the dot areas in the diagram.

> Breathe slowly and deeply. Note the sensations at each point.

EXERCISE

RELEASING SCALP AND JAW MUSCLES WITH MASSAGE

In many headaches, the muscles of the face, jaw, and scalp will tighten, worsening the intensity of the headache or even triggering more headaches. In this exercise, we use dynamic motion and pressure to release these muscles.

> Take your index and third fingers and find your chewing/jaw muscles. Place your fingers in the center of this muscle and make small circles. If you can feel any tightness, pause and apply continuous pressure. Try to get to know these muscles. Is one side tighter than the other? Fuller than the other?

> Apply firm pressure to the center of your jaw muscles. Now open your mouth slowly, maintaining that pressure. Open your mouth as wide as you can, all while maintaining that pressure.

> Repeat three to five times and shift the placement of your fingers to other spots on that muscle while opening your jaw slowly.

> Now find your temporalis muscle. Take the fingertips of your index through pinky fingers. Place them cupping over the tops of your ears, with the fingertips firmly pressing into your scalp.

While applying pressure, drag your fingers up to the top of your head in a slow gradual motion. Feel the large muscles begin to release. Repeat three to five times.

If it is tolerable, open your mouth slowly as you drag your fingers up from your ears to the top of your head. Apply continuous pressure.

Repeat the movement of releasing your temporalis muscle while opening your jaw three to five times.

CHAPTER 8

Brain Fog, Dysautonomia, and Other Nervous System Imbalances

Brain fog made it very hard to focus in school, and concentrate, and get work done. It was like I couldn't think. I've never had that problem before. I'm an intelligent person, I always made really good grades, it came naturally. But all of a sudden it was like my brain just would not work for me. That was a very new and challenging experience.

What You Will Learn in This Chapter:

- The neuroscience of memory
- The causes of brain fog, and how to get evaluated
- Tools and strategies for maximizing neuroplasticity and neurologic recovery
- An overview of dysautonomia and postural orthostatic tachycardia syndrome (POTS), a common problem in long illness
- Tips and tools for reducing the debilitating symptoms of dysautonomia
- Nervous system imbalances in general
- Testing and lifestyle changes

Fumbling for the right words is frustrating. *Why do I feel this way? It didn't used to be this hard to think.*

Memory problems and brain fog, which are distressing symptoms of long illness for many people, make everyday functioning more difficult. Brain fog comes and goes. It can change day to day, even hour to hour. Its episodic nature can make it hard to capture, treat, and study. When many people talk to their practitioners, the brain fog they describe often gets brushed aside. But brain fog is real.

As you read this chapter, you may notice that you experience more brain fog. When we focus our attention on it, brain fog can amplify. This is okay. If it becomes too intense, take a break. But if you can, take notice of this feeling and keep going. Brain fog may be showing up while you read about it so that it can be addressed more fully. See how it shifts and changes. Try the tools provided here and see which ones clear away some fog.

What Is Memory?

Think about a wonderful event from your childhood. Even years later, you probably still recall details about what you saw and how you felt. How does an experience become a memory?

It starts with paying attention. If we can't focus on something, the brain can't understand and store it. Poor sleep, anxiety, depression, trauma, and inflammation can all worsen attention, as can a busy mind full of thoughts and worries. What we think is a memory problem is really an attention problem.

Once you've paid attention to and taken in an experience, it is stored as a short-term memory. You can remember what you ate for breakfast this morning but not a week ago because your mind kept that breakfast memory in short-term storage but didn't feel that it was important enough to remember over the long term. More short-term memories are forgotten than transferred to long-term storage. Memories that get prioritized are often those associated with new experiences or those with emotional significance.

Your state of mind plays a big role in whether a short-term memory goes into long-term storage. The brain can't prioritize thinking and learning if it feels like there is an imminent threat or something more important to pay attention to. Sleep has also been shown to affect memory. When you sleep badly, your brain simply doesn't have the bandwidth for extra learning.

When you try to remember something, you have to retrieve that memory out of storage. Your memories are scattered strategically throughout the brain, not stored all in one place. Finding where the memory is stored requires some degree of organization. When this search for the memory is slow, we call it a problem with *processing speed*. There is some evidence that processing speed can be reduced by a number of factors common in long illness, including increased inflammation and depression.

In most cases, brain fog impairs attention and usually affects processing speed too. Brain fog is just like foggy weather: fog covers up details and slows everything down.

What Is Brain Fog?

Brain fog broadly describes a problem with attention and memory. The details, though, vary from person to person: some have problems with multitasking, others respond slowly to questions, and still others are unable to pay attention at work or school. Improving brain fog requires a holistic approach. Why? Because brain fog is a symptom. It appears to be the brain's reaction to imbalance, overload, and inflammation. We need to target the roots of the problem—or problems.

We don't yet understand why some people's brains are more predisposed to developing fog. For some, it's their mind's way of telling them they are overloaded. For others, brain fog can be caused by something as specific as a food they have eaten. Here are some common causes of brain fog.

Fatigue	Gut problems	Concussions	Dehydration
Inflammation	Trauma	Depression	Poor sleep
Pain	Migraines	Anxiety	Food sensitivities
Medication effects	Hormone imbalances	ADHD	Blood pressure changes
	Vitamin deficiencies	Trauma	

Can you connect any of these problems with your brain fog? You may want to write them down in your journal.

Some of these causes of brain fog already have dedicated chapters in this book. Referring back to those chapters can help you target the underlying problem and lift the fog. Let's take a look at some of the rest of them:

ADHD and attention problems	Some of the symptoms of ADHD (attention deficit/hyperactivity disorder) can masquerade as brain fog, including feeling "spacey," difficulty multitasking, and difficulty keeping track of schedules. To be evaluated for a problem with attention, talk to your primary care practitioner.
Blood pressure	Blood pressure that is too high, too low, or changing suddenly can cause brain fog. Talk to your primary practitioner about purchasing a home blood pressure cuff to record your measurements at home. If rapid blood pressure shifts are a problem for you, read the section here on dysautonomia.
Mast cell activation syndrome (MCAS)	MCAS is a problem with the allergy response system in the body and can involve symptoms like flushing, abdominal discomfort, brain fog, and problems with low blood pressure. Diagnosis involves lab tests ordered by your primary practitioner or allergist and is often supplemented with testing for dysautonomia.
Medication side effects	Many medications, including those to treat sleep disorders or blood pressure, can cause brain fog. Review your medication list with your primary practitioner to see if a medication could be contributing to the problem.
Vitamin deficiencies	Several vitamin deficiencies can manifest as brain fog, including low levels of vitamin B_{12}, vitamin D, or iron. Many of these we can test for easily and inexpensively. Ask your practitioner if screening for vitamin deficiencies is right for you.
Concussions	Concussions affect whole networks in the brain, not just the area of injury. If you have been concussed, your brain may often need more care and attention to factors like sleep and nutrition and be less forgiving of all-nighters or skipping a meal than it was prior to injury.
Dehydration	The brain is mostly water and is sensitive to fluid levels in your body. We know that even small amounts of dehydration can affect learning and thinking. Even a 1 percent loss of water from the body can result in brain fog. (Chapter 15 can help you optimize your hydration.)
Hormones	Hormonal changes that occur before, during, and after menopause can cause brain fog. Hormone fluctuations around periods can also cause mood changes and brain fog. The same is true for low testosterone in men. Other hormones, like thyroid hormones, are also implicated in causing brain fog. Talk to your primary practitioner about whether hormones could be contributing to your fog.

Brain Fog Versus Dementia

For the most part, brain fog and dementia are very different conditions.

Think of the brain as a computer. As we said earlier, brain fog is a problem with the software: the fog slows everything down and makes the software slow to run, but the structure of the brain, the hardware, is okay.

Dementia, on the other hand, is a hardware problem. In dementia, the brain gets more and more damaged over time, and thinking and memory become impaired as a result. We worry about dementia when someone isn't just having difficulty thinking quickly or paying attention, but also seems unable to manage their usual activities of daily living and may be inadvertently putting themselves in unsafe situations. This is different from the normal memory changes with aging. In healthy brain aging, people can be expected to have a harder time remembering details or names, but this doesn't impair their ability to take care of themselves.

If you answer "yes" to any of the following questions, you can use that as a jumping-off point in speaking with your primary care practitioner or neurologist about a memory evaluation.

Are you getting lost in familiar places?

Are you leaving the stove on, leaving the door open, or raising other safety concerns at home with your actions as a result of memory lapses?

Have memory problems prevented you from working, socializing, or feeling safe?

Is it consistently difficult for you to follow the flow of conversations?

Is your memory loss noticeably impairing your ability to participate in the usual activities of your life?

Memory and Thinking Evaluations

A memory evaluation usually starts with completing a screening worksheet in your primary practitioner's office in order to give them a sense of how your thinking and memory are working. Depending on your results, your primary practitioner can consider expanding the testing to get more information.

Expanded testing is done by specialized psychologists who perform neuropsychological (also known as neurocognitive) testing. This memory testing is usually several hours long. It looks at many areas of thinking, learning, and memory. Once this test is completed, you and your care team will have a fuller sense of your thinking and memory problems. The results of these tests may change over time and can be repeated at one- to three-year intervals (or more frequently depending on your practitioner's recommendation).

> *Some days, for no reason, my brain feels like it is made of sludge. My thoughts feel like they just can't get out. I'm a very well organized, efficient person. It feels so sudden, like I'm cognitively moving through quicksand.*

Brain Fog Clearing and Memory Optimizing Tool Kit

Once you have targeted underlying causes and understand your unique brain's strengths and weaknesses, you can design an integrative medicine recovery plan. Some large medical centers offer *cognitive rehabilitation*, a type of rehab specifically aimed at strengthening thinking and memory. If this service is not available where you live, your health care team can design a recovery program for you.

Maximizing Neuroplasticity

Adult brains can develop new capacities and make new connections, even in the face of illness. This is called *neuroplasticity*.

Neurologic recovery looks different depending on what is happening with your unique brain. With the right brain training and environment, you can clear the fog and harness your neuroplasticity. Even just one activity a day is a great place to start and likely to help your brain grow. Here are some tools and ideas to help:

Play cards. Start with a simple game like War, then try Go Fish or Uno. Even simple games keep your brain engaged.

Work with numbers. Try simple calculations in your head. Try sudoku or balance your checkbook.

Enhance your spatial reasoning. Assemble puzzles, draw a map of your neighborhood from memory, or sketch the fruit on your table.

Strengthen your memory. Try to recall meaningful life events. Tell them to a friend or write them down. Push yourself to remember as many details as possible.

Involve all the senses. Seek out experiences that bring together sound, taste, smell, sight, and touch. For instance, go to a farmers' market or interactive museum.

Try something new. New activities create new networks in the brain. Go to another part of your neighborhood or town and explore, pick up a few words in a new language, or listen to new music.

Get some exercise. Exercise enhances neuroplasticity, prevents cognitive decline, and supports thinking. (Check out Chapter 19 for more details.)

Socialize. Loneliness is hard on the brain. When you socialize, you are using multiple parts of your brain to process language and pick up on social cues. From research, we know that socializing protects against dementia. There are lots of reasons why socializing can be hard with a long illness. Thinking of it as a tool for neurologic recovery can motivate you to find a way to socialize that works for you.

Stay hydrated and eat a MIND diet (see next section).

Go outside. Getting connected to nature has an anti-inflammatory effect and reduces stress hormones. Being in nature can strengthen memory and attention. The more time you spend in nature, and the more removed it is from urban settings, the better. "Forest bathing," spending time immersed in a forest or lush park, is a great way to feel the full effects of "nature medicine." Your time outdoors doesn't have to be an active time. Lying or sitting in any green space can be medicine. If a green space outdoors is not immediately available to you, just having indoor plants can help regulate your nervous system and clear brain fog.

Practice mindfulness. Mindfulness can be a powerful tool for balancing your nervous system and clearing the mind. Try out the mindfulness exercise in the next section and read Chapter 16 to learn more about stress and mindfulness.

Biomedicine. Currently, we don't have medications approved to target brain fog as a primary symptom. It can be frustrating to be offered so few options for treatment. In our clinics, we use several low-risk biomedicines off-label, including medications that are used in other memory conditions and low-dose naltrexone (discussed in Chapters 4 and 5). We use antidepressant medications with someone who also has anxiety or depression, primarily for their anti-inflammatory benefit.

Brain Protection with the MIND Diet

Diet nourishes your brain. The Mediterranean-DASH Intervention for Neurodegenerative Delay (MIND) diet has been shown in studies to improve brain health, slow cognitive decline, and protect brain functioning. Brains seem to age more slowly on this diet. That was not true for the Mediterranean diet alone. The MIND diet is currently considered the most protective diet for brain health and recovery.

The MIND diet follows the principles of other anti-inflammatory diets and recommends eating specific foods that we know improve brain health, like lots of leafy greens and berries (which can be purchased frozen to reduce cost). Olive oil is the primary oil recommended because it is neuroprotective and enhances thinking.

The guidelines for the MIND diet are pretty straightforward:

Enjoy daily: Dark leafy greens, other vegetables (eat the rainbow), whole grains, nuts, olive oil, beans

Enjoy at least twice a week: Berries, poultry
Enjoy at least once a week: Fish
Limit: Butter, cheese, red meat, sugary foods, fried foods

Some practitioners include limited amounts of red wine in this diet. If you choose to include wine, limit it to no more than one glass per day.

Other Diets

Certain food-related conditions, like a sensitivity or allergy to gluten, can cause brain fog. Your body's unique relationship to food may require a deeper investigation.

We do not routinely recommend ordering food allergy tests, because current tests are not accurate enough. They are often costly without producing clear evidence of true allergy. For people with brain fog that isn't improving, we often recommend an elimination diet paired with a food journal. In this approach, you cut back potentially allergic foods and then add them back slowly. With each food you add back, you can ask yourself: How is my brain fog after cutting out this food? See our discussion in Chapters 17 and 18 to learn more about food journaling and elimination diets.

Clearing Brain Fog Exercise

Mindfulness and visualization can be useful tools in clearing or shifting brain fog. We also know that deep breaths strengthen the rest-and-digest parasympathetic nervous system and can have anti-inflammatory benefits. This breathwork exercise can reduce brain fog on many levels. Follow these instructions (or record the exercise on your phone and play it back for yourself):

Find a quiet place to sit or lie down or to settle in whatever position is comfortable for your body. Set a five-minute timer. Close your eyes.
Notice the current weather in your mind. Is there fog there? How thick is it? Does it have a quality, temperature, or texture? Take a moment to

simply notice it. Allow for any feelings around the fog to be with you too. If you can, take a moment to acknowledge these feelings. Keep breathing and noticing.

Take a deep breath in, and on the exhale begin to breathe out the fog. Take long, slow, deep breaths. With each exhale, notice more of the fog clearing. It may evaporate, float away, or simply move out of your mind. It may travel back to the clouds, or land on the soil.

As the fog shifts, notice if anything else moves with it, like anxiety, worry, or pain. Allow anything else that doesn't serve you to also be cleared.

Continue deep breathing and clearing on the exhale for five minutes.

When the time is up, you can keep going or stop. Notice the weather of your mind again. Notice the relaxation and any clearing that occurred in your body. Allow yourself some restful time for several minutes to just *be*.

You can return to this exercise anytime. Whether you're in a meeting or out on a walk, you can use deep breaths to help clear brain fog.

Autonomic Nervous System Dysfunction and Dysautonomia

Before getting sick, I had a stable resting heart rate in the 60s. Then it was like, "What is my body doing to me?" My heart rate would go up and stay there, leaving me tired and out of breath. It was scary, I was not used to my body not obeying me. Now I have learned to think less about the numbers and focus on how I feel. I am being patient with myself and learning how to listen to what my body needs. It's not easy, but it is getting more manageable.

Long illness can wear down the body's electrical system, called the *autonomic nervous system* (ANS). The result can be lightheadedness, fatigue, and brain fog. The ANS feeds and balances the body through two branches: the fight-or-flight sympathetic nervous system and the rest-and-digest parasympathetic nervous system. Think of the two branches of the ANS as the accelerator and brake pedals on a car. If they are in balance, your body functions at the right speed. If they aren't, your body can go too fast or too slow, or even crash. Let's review some of the functions of the two systems:

Fight-or-Flight Sympathetic Nervous System	Rest-and-Digest Parasympathetic Nervous System
Heartbeat increases	Heartbeat slows
Digestion is slowed	Digestion is stimulated
Blood pressure increases	Blood pressure decreases
Intestines move slower	Intestines move faster
Anxiety increases	Anxiety decreases
Stress hormones increase	Stress hormones decrease
Body breaks down and releases energy (catabolic)	Body restores and conserves energy (anabolic)

Both branches of the autonomic nervous system keep the body running smoothly. When this system is slightly off-balance, people can experience difficulty relaxing, brain fog, and occasional dizziness when they stand. Practitioners rarely offer testing for those having these symptoms, but they are still distressing. More severe damage to the autonomic system will sustain rapid shifts in heart rate and blood pressure. Testing can lead to a diagnosis of *dysautonomia*, which simply refers to a group of medical conditions caused by problems with the autonomic nervous system.

There are many different dysautonomia syndromes. Postural orthostatic tachycardia syndrome (POTS) and neurocardiogenic syncope (aka vasovagal syncope or fainting spells) are the two most common. POTS is common in teenagers, and many experience improvement in their symptoms with age. However, POTS can happen at any age, and the impairment experienced in this condition can be serious. Dysautonomia also is a common secondary symptom of other conditions or occurs because of an underlying condition—most commonly multiple sclerosis, diabetes, celiac disease, Parkinson's, and rheumatological disease. Treatment of the underlying disease in these cases can be helpful with symptoms.

Here is a list of common symptoms of dysautonomia. Experiencing these symptoms doesn't necessarily mean that you have damage to your nervous system. But they can provide a jumping-off point to discuss possible testing with your health care team. Many people with symptoms of dysautonomia experience years of diagnostic delay, so tell your health care team and ask to see a specialist early, as it can take time to get appointments with these experts.

Lightheadedness
Feeling like you are going to pass out
Tachycardia/high heart rate, especially on standing
Low blood pressure
Symptoms when you stand quickly or change positions
Palpitations
Abnormal sweating
Fatigue
Exercise intolerance
Brain fog
Constipation and other GI distress
Temperature sensitivity

Dysautonomia can result from a host of underlying conditions. It can come from a problem in your central nervous system (brain/spinal cord) or peripheral nervous system (the nerve network that activates your body outside of your brain and spinal cord). It can occur in post-infectious syndromes, autoimmune diseases, severe medical illnesses, pregnancy, and head injury. Some diseases have a directly toxic effect on the nerves. For example, the high sugar levels experienced by those with diabetes are damaging to the nerves. Inflammation and autoimmunity also underlie many cases of dysautonomia. Chronic stress, trauma, anxiety, and depression can upset the balance of the nervous system. There is testing that can diagnose these conditions and pinpoint which part of the nervous system is struggling.

How Do We Test for Dysautonomia?

Autonomic testing is done by specialists, usually a cardiologist or a neurologist. The common tests are:

Tilt table test	While you're lying on a table that can shift up and down, your heart rate and blood pressure are monitored to see how they adjust to different positions. This is the main test used to diagnose these conditions.
Sweat test	Checking the amount that your body sweats on the surface is a way to evaluate your ANS.
Electrocardiogram	A screening electrocardiogram (ECG) can rule out structural heart problems.
Blood tests	Blood tests may include a comprehensive metabolic panel, thyroid studies, vitamin studies (vitamins D and B_{12}), and tests to determine catecholamine levels (substances in your body that regulate blood pressure and heart rate).
Biopsies	In some cases a small piece of skin is removed to look at the health of the smallest nerves.

Mast Cell Activation Syndrome (MCAS)

Mast cell activation syndrome is a potential cause of POTS syndrome in some people. MCAS often goes undiagnosed owing to lack of awareness around this illness and difficulty with testing. In addition to dysautonomia, the symptoms include widespread allergies and sensitivities with systemic inflammation and skin problems like cysts and rashes. This illness is a dysfunction of the mast cells in the body, which mediate allergic reactions and inflammation. Mast cells can also impact blood vessel constriction or dilation. When not functioning properly, they can cause rapid changes in blood pressure, as we see in dysautonomia. MCAS is a treatable condition. To get a diagnosis you should seek the care of an allergy specialist. The testing and treatment are complicated, and allergists are more likely to provide you with accurate testing and appropriate management.

Treatment

Whether or not you have a formal diagnosis of dysautonomia, there are treatments that can strengthen your autonomic nervous system, reduce your cortisol levels, and bring more balance to your ANS. Chronic illness, inflammation, trauma, depression, and anxiety can all rev up the sympathetic nervous system. Here are a few of our key recommendations for rebalancing.

Hydrate	Lightheadedness and brain fog can often improve significantly if you are able to maintain adequate hydration. The targets are 2.7 liters per day for women and 3.7 liters per day for men. We often set higher targets for people with dysautonomia. Talk to your primary practitioner about your optimal fluid goals.
Exercise	Exercise strengthens your heart and ANS. Ask your primary practitioner about a referral to physical therapy if you are uncertain about how to exercise safely. It is crucial to make your transitions from lying down to sitting and from sitting to standing as slow as necessary. Try the isometric contraction exercise here before making big transitions. Give your body time to adjust to each new position.
Increase salt	Increasing your salt intake can increase your blood pressure and reduce lightheadedness. This is not an appropriate change for most people, especially those with high blood pressure and other health conditions, so be sure to discuss with your primary care practitioner.
Eat smaller meals	Large meals can be taxing on the nervous system. You are less likely to be fatigued and lightheaded after eating a smaller meal.
Compression	Try wearing compression socks and talk to your practitioner about whether an abdominal binder would be appropriate to keep blood from pooling in your legs.
Medications	There are medications for treating dysautonomia that work on heart rate and regulate blood pressure. For those with MCAS, the treatment is allergy medications. Medications need to be prescribed and monitored by skilled practitioners, and they are almost always taken in conjunction with lifestyle treatments.
Anti-inflammatory diet	Anti-inflammatory foods give your body the fuel it needs to recalibrate and strengthen your nervous system. See Chapter 18.

EXERCISE

ISOMETRIC CONTRACTION

Try this exercise first thing in the morning while lying in bed, or anytime you are about to change positions. It can also be helpful if you have been standing for a long period of time. The exercise gets the blood circulating and can reduce dizziness.

Contract and scrunch your toes tightly, hold for ten seconds, then release.

Move up to your calves. Squeeze firmly, hold for ten seconds, then release.

Move upward, squeezing, holding, and releasing. Remember to include your abdominal muscles, pelvic floor, arms, and facial muscles.

When you have completed one cycle, breathe deeply for three breaths. Move slowly into your next position, like sitting or standing up.

CHAPTER 9

Digestion Disruption

It is rare to meet someone with long illness who hasn't experienced disruption to their digestion. This happens because your gastrointestinal tract is intimately linked to your immune and nervous systems as well as sensitive to inflammation. Your digestion is often at the core of your overall health, both physical and mental. There is a reason they call it a "gut feeling." Your *enteric nervous system*, the nervous system in your gut, contains more neurons than your spinal cord, and it produces the majority of your body's serotonin, the "happiness" molecule that regulates your mood.

What You Will Learn in This Chapter:

- An overview of gut health and the power of your body's microbiome
- Tips for treating common problems arising in the gut: reflux, inflammatory bowel disease, irritable bowel disease, leaky gut, and small intestinal bacterial overgrowth
- Integrative tools to balance and support gut health

What Is Your Gut?

Your gastrointestinal tract (your gut, or GI tract) starts at your mouth and ends at your rear end, to put it politely. As soon as food hits your mouth, digestion starts. Your mouth, esophagus, stomach, small intestine, pancreas, large intestine, and anus make up your GI tract. At each step, chemical reactions and mechanical steps allow for the extraction of nutrients from whatever you put in your mouth. But your gut doesn't work alone. It gets help from your microbiome, the trillions of microbes that live in harmony with your body and help you thrive.

Microbiome Basics

Your body is made up of about 30 trillion human cells and 39 trillion microbes. Communities of bacteria, archaea, viruses, and fungi (collectively, *microbiota*, or microbes) living in and on your body make up your unique *microbiome*. They are essential to your ability to fight illness, reduce inflammation, regulate mood, and digest food. A big part of the microbiome lives in your gut. Your gut microbiome weighs about two kilograms (4.5 pounds) and is bigger than your brain.

Without your microbiome, you wouldn't be you; it is uniquely yours. Gut microbiota affect many areas of your health by helping your immune system develop, defending your body against pathogens (for example, bad microbes), making vitamins, absorbing nutrients, helping you store fat, facilitating your metabolism, controlling your appetite, and influencing your moods. Your microbiome composition also influences your response to medications.

Part of your microbiome is genetic, but environmental factors like diet and medications determine the makeup of most of your microbiome. Although microbiomes are unique, we also see patterns, referred to as microbiome profiles, in patients with different conditions ranging from liver fibrosis to Crohn's disease. Analysis of the microbiome can help practitioners diagnose and formulate treatment plans for many diseases, including cancer, and can even help predict the risk of diseases like type 2 diabetes.

Your diet and medications have a strong influence on the composition of your gut microbiota. So what does your gut need to thrive? It is simple: your gut needs for you to eat food (which has prebiotics) to feed the good bacteria (probiotics) and to avoid things that can cause *dysbiosis*, an imbalance of microbes that changes your health.

It's All Connected

Your gut and your brain are connected from the start of life. Your stomach really does have a mind of its own. The enteric nervous system helps change blood flow to the gut, assists in food digestion, modulates hormone levels, eliminates toxins, and controls the passage of food through your gut. The enteric nervous system can act entirely on its own without the brain, but surprisingly, 90 percent of the communication is from the gut to the brain. This communication is referred to as the *microbiome-gut-brain axis*.

A whopping 70 percent of your immune system lives in your gut alongside your microbiome. Your microbiome also communicates with your brain through its effects on the immune cells in your gut, which make a wide range of chemicals that affect the brain. Anything that kills the flora in your gut can reduce immune support. This is particularly worrisome in people who have chronic illness and are exposed to repeated sickness and injury.

How Does Your Microbiome Affect Your Mood?

We now know that our gut microbiome helps make neurotransmitters, like serotonin, that work all over our body. Research over the last ten years has found that different microbe populations in the gut are associated with different moods, such as depression and anxiety. The moods of mice with depression and anxiety improve when they are fed particular strains of bacteria.

Research in humans has shown that ingestion of certain psychobiotics (probiotics aimed at addressing mood issues) can reduce stress hormones, improve anxiety, depression, and worry, make emotional processing healthier, and help prevent postpartum depression and anxiety. We expect more specific recommendations in the future for improving mood and cognitive symptoms using dietary modifications and supplementation with evidence-based psychobiotics.

We also know that people who have gastrointestinal issues are more likely to experience depression and anxiety than other people. We used to think depression caused changes in gut health, but we are learning that it is likely the other way around. For example, cognitive behavior therapy and antidepressants—treatments for the brain—have been shown to be helpful in reducing GI symptoms in some patients by calming down nerve cells in the gut.

What Is Bad for Your Gut?

Limit added sugars, artificial sweeteners, and refined carbohydrates. Reduce your red meat consumption, cut out processed meats, and opt for nonconventionally farmed animal products when possible. Look out for added preservatives and additives, as they can disrupt the gut on multiple levels. Take only the medications and supplements you actually need. Reduce your exposure to toxins. Eating a diverse diet exposes you to more microbes, so try new foods and incorporate them into your routine. A limited diet limits microbiome diversity. Stress is also bad for your gut, so practicing skills that reduce stress can help.

Should You Avoid Antibiotics?

After a course of antibiotics, it can take up to a year to repopulate your gut flora. Some people need to be on antibiotics often or continuously because of underlying conditions. Antibiotics from our food supply (in meat from animals who have been treated with antibiotics) can also disrupt your microbiome.

Take antibiotics when you need them, but pair them with a change in your diet along with probiotic supplements. Taking probiotics paired with antibiotics can prevent and treat antibiotic-associated diarrhea and it can also reduce your chance of *Clostridium difficile* infection, which occurs when your microbiome is weakened and these bacteria take over.

There are many ways in which long illness can affect your GI system, as well as many theories about what could be causing your underlying gut issues. Let's talk about the more common ones we are asked about.

Reflux

The most common gut-related symptom in long illness is gastroesophageal reflux disease (GERD), which arises from problems with the upper gastrointestinal tract. Reflux is common and easily managed, but it can also be a sign of something more serious. As with most symptoms, the first step is to talk to your primary practitioner to make sure you receive appropriate screening for other potential causes.

For treatment of reflux, we use a mix of lifestyle medicine, natural products, and biomedical approaches. Common food triggers are alcohol, chocolate, coffee, caffeine, dairy, fatty foods, spicy foods, citrus, tomatoes, mint, and soda. Modifying your diet by avoiding these foods, at least in the short term while your esophagus heals, is usually the first step. An elimination diet of these foods with a symptom journal can be a good way to start eliminating one food at a time and noticing whether your symptoms improve. (See page 260 for more information on the elimination diet.)

Here are a few easy lifestyle changes to lessen symptoms:

Avoid drinking more than a few sips of fluids with meals.

Allow at least two hours for digestion between dinner and bedtime.

Talk to your doctor about raising your head at night by putting blocks underneath the legs at the head of your bed. Avoid adding extra pillows to raise your head, as this may compress your stomach more and increase reflux symptoms.

Improve your digestion by exercising, but avoid vigorous exercise directly after meals.

Increase your intake of fiber.

Many patients with reflux explore natural products for their symptoms, including deglycyrrhizinated licorice, marshmallow root, slippery elm, chamomile, and melatonin. These are generally safe, but as with any new treatment, it's important to talk with your primary practitioners or gastro-enterologist before starting on them.

Relaxation techniques, like mindfulness, hypnotherapy, and biofeed-back, have also been shown in studies to improve reflux symptoms, since they work on regulating the nervous system. Acupuncture can also be effective. Emotional stress can reduce saliva and increase reflux symptoms, so addressing any stress or psychological roots of your reflux can be an important part of addressing this symptom if it isn't getting better using other techniques. Many people use medications like proton pump inhibi-tors. They can cause vitamin deficiencies and increase your risk of certain infections and fractures, however, so always consider alternative options first.

What Are IBS and IBD?

Irritable bowel syndrome (IBS) and inflammatory bowel disease (IBD) sound similar but are very different.

IBS, a functional gastrointestinal disorder, is a disturbance between the gut and the brain that affects bowel function and doesn't have a great medi-cal explanation. Movement in the colon is irregular in people who experi-ence IBS. Many people who experience symptoms like chronic abdominal pain, cramping, belching, or bloating related to defecation are diagnosed with IBS. This disorder is more common in people who have chronic fatigue syndrome, GERD, depression, anxiety, or fibromyalgia. Many people with IBS have experienced severe food poisoning in the past. The disease flares up in late adolescence or early adulthood and is usually associated with stress. There are usually no findings of IBS using endoscopy because it does not cause inflammation of the gastrointestinal tissue.

Evidence-based treatment includes education, medications, cognitive behavioral therapy, stress reduction, and relaxation techniques, as well as integrative techniques like gut-directed hypnotherapy. Read in the next sec-tion about the FODMaP diet and see page 260 for information on an elimi-nation diet, which can have a big impact on IBS symptoms.

Inflammatory bowel disease, an inflammation of the intestines, includes Crohn's disease and ulcerative colitis. IBD is largely genetic, but flares and quality of life are greatly affected by lifestyle habits. It is diagnosed with biopsies and imaging. The inflammatory damage to the GI tract can be permanent and significant and may require surgery to correct. Patients with IBD have an increased risk for colon cancer and should be under the supervision of a gastroenterologist. Many changes that people make for IBS can be helpful for those with IBD, but medications that target the immune system are often needed in IBD to prevent severe complications.

Treating IBS with Diet

The FODMaP diet cuts out Fermentable Oligosaccharides, Disaccharides, Monosaccharides, and Polyols. These fermentable carbohydrates are poorly absorbed by your digestive system and will sit in your gut causing trouble: bloating, gas, pain. For those with irritable bowel syndrome or similar symptoms, this diet might be helpful. It works best in people whose predominant symptom is diarrhea, although some improvement has been seen in people who have constipation-predominant symptoms. Abdominal pain, bloating, flatulence, and diarrhea improve in people who cut down on these foods. The symptoms depend on the amount of the food consumed. This means that eating a single cherry might be okay, but eating a cup of cherries will trigger your symptoms.

We recommend reviewing your food diary and noting if any of the foods you eat are high-FODMaP sources. There are more extensive lists online, but the table here is a good place to start. Cut down on these foods for a week and see if you notice a difference. Talk to your practitioner about your experience to see if you should try an elimination and reintroduction FODMaP diet or if just cutting back on high-FODMaP foods is enough to keep your symptoms under control. Sometimes just knowing more about your IBS food triggers and eating a more plant-based anti-inflammatory diet can help reduce symptoms. This table provides the basics; see the resources section at the back of the book for more.

Fermentable Sugar	Class of Sugar	Food Sources
Oligosaccharides	Fructans and galactans	Onion, garlic, beans, broccoli, asparagus, large amounts of wheat or rye (as in bread), pasta, chickpeas, baked beans, lentils, watermelon, peaches
Disaccharides	Lactose	Milk, ice cream, yogurt, soft and fresh cheeses
Monosaccharides	Fructose	Mainly fruits or added fructose, as in apples, pears, peaches, honey, fructose, high-fructose corn syrup, fruit juices, dried fruit
Polyol sweeteners	Sorbitol	Sorbitol, isomalt, mannitol, xylitol, and other sources ending in "-ol" found on nutrition labels; also avocados, mushrooms, apples, cherries, pears

The FODMaP diet is highly restrictive, and many of the foods it eliminates are healthy and beneficial to your gut microbiome. It decreases the diversity of your gut microbiome, which can lead to many other issues. If you do not have IBS symptoms, or if the FODMaP diet is not recommended by your practitioner, you should not try it. If it is recommended for you, follow the FODMaP diet only temporarily, until you can identify the foods and amounts that trigger your symptoms.

You are cutting out a lot of processed foods when you limit the sugars often added to these foods. Many people also report that their symptoms go away on a gluten-free diet, which cuts out about 50 percent of the typical FODMaP sources. It is the fructans they cut out, however, that were causing symptoms, not the gluten. Others discover that a certain sugar type always triggers their issues. Some find that they can continue to eat their favorite foods, just in lower amounts.

What Is Leaky Gut?

Your body engages in a very complex process to extract nutrients from the food you eat while also keeping microbes, toxic digestive metabolites, bacterial toxins, and small molecules inside your gut. The cells of the gut epithelium (the lining of your GI tract) are tightly connected, like superglue.

But this security system is not as impenetrable as we once thought. Studies have shown that, for multiple reasons, including genetic differences, certain bacterial pathogens and high blood sugar can make it easier for bacteria to come into the intestine. And sometimes increased permeability triggers autoimmune-like symptoms and systemic inflammation. There is still much to learn, however, before this evidence can be used in treating long illnesses. In fact, many practitioners and scientists have been skeptical of leaky gut—or to be more technically correct, increased intestinal permeability.

That said, permeability is important to consider if you have a long illness. Your relatively greater exposure to medications, treatments, stress, and pathogens leaves your gut barrier more at risk for inflammation and possibly increased permeability to pathogenic materials. Several companies offer tests that will give you more information about your gut health. Some tests offered by practitioners look for levels of indigestible sugars in your urine. These tests might provide some interesting information, but the results won't change your practitioners' recommendations. The evidence is clear that reducing processed-food intake and adopting an anti-inflammatory diet is the best way to improve problems of intestinal permeability.

There is evidence that L-glutamine supplementation and marshmallow tea may help. Several other natural products can help with abdominal pain, cramping, gas, and other symptoms. (See Chapter 21 on natural products.)

What About Yeast?

Yeast is normal in the gut. In fact, some probiotics contain strains of yeast. Some people can have an overgrowth of yeast in connection with diseases like IBD or because they are immunosuppressed. Yeast can also overgrow in the vagina, especially after a disruption to the microbiome (as when you take antibiotics). The overgrowth of Candida yeast can disrupt your epithelial gut barrier. Sometimes these conditions can be treated with antifungals.

Some practitioners believe that stopping sugars and avoiding dairy and gluten can help. You also can try low-lactose and gluten-free diets to see if they reduce symptoms from yeast overgrowth.

We don't have the evidence to recommend yeast cleanse products or other yeast-reducing supplements. Work with your primary practitioner to understand whether yeast is a problem for you and what dietary changes could shift your microbiome.

What If You Have Microbe Overgrowth?

Some people have an overgrowth of microbes that make too much gas. If you are overeating or not digesting your food well, nutrients that are normally absorbed in the small intestine pass into the large intestine, where they cause gas, bloating, distention, pain, or diarrhea. This may be small intestine bacterial overgrowth (SIBO) or intestinal methanogen (methane-producing organism) overgrowth (IMO). Microbial overgrowth underlies many cases of IBS but often goes undiagnosed.

Breath tests are used to determine if you have SIBO or IMO. Your practitioner can order the test, which is available either in person or by mail. Your practitioner may recommend invasive testing (such as endoscopy) in some situations to help diagnose these conditions.

The treatment for proven overgrowth is antibiotics. While some practitioners might suggest that you try antibiotics without testing for overgrowth, we suggest having a test for SIBO/IMO first. Some overgrowth can be treated effectively with diet and lifestyle modifications and treatment of the underlying cause of your microbe overgrowth. You should work with your practitioner to optimize lifestyle changes and treat known disease first. A low-FODMaP diet can be helpful for some people.

Microbe overgrowth is more common in certain conditions that interfere with the proper functioning of your gastrointestinal tract. These include diabetes, inflammatory bowel disease, opiate use, aging, small bowel diverticulosis, HIV, CVID, IgA deficiency, cirrhosis, and pancreatic insufficiency, to name a new. If possible, treatment of the underlying cause is essential to prevent recurrence and avoid multiple rounds of antibiotics.

What Is Fecal Transplantation? Can It Help You?

Fecal transplant was developed to treat a severe infection of the gut called *Clostridium difficile* (C. diff). This infection can arise when people are on antibiotics, which wipe out good bacteria and allow C. diff to overgrow. C. diff can be not only hard to treat but deadly.

Enter fecal microbiota transplants (FMTs). The basic concept is that fecal material is taken from a healthy donor and transferred into the GI tract of a sick person, with the hope that microbial diversity will be increased and a healthier microbiome established.

FMT is currently permitted for C. diff treatment only. The good news is that research is ongoing on the role of FMT in treating long illnesses thought to include a disrupted microbiome, including ME/CFS, irritable bowel syndrome, inflammatory bowel syndrome, and depression. It is likely that in the future FMT and other more individually tailored microbiota editing techniques will be available. The evidence thus far is promising for some conditions, but more clinical trials are needed.

What About Prebiotics and Probiotics?

Prebiotics are plant-based fibers that keep the gut microbiome healthy; they feed your microbiome. You need at least thirty grams of fiber a day, which most of us don't get regularly. For those dealing with an underlying illness, getting enough fiber and eating healthy foods can be difficult. At the same time, getting adequate fiber and eating a healthy diet can make GI symptoms worse for some people.

Prebiotics help with the absorption of minerals like iron, magnesium, and calcium, and they help your immune system fight disease better. Eat a diverse range of the prebiotic types listed in this table to give your microbiome a bigger menu to choose from.

Table 1

FOODS HIGH IN FIBER

High-Fiber Food Groups	Examples
Legumes	Navy beans, lentils, green peas
Whole grains	Rolled oats, oatmeal, oat bran, whole wheat
Fruit	Avocados, passion fruit, pears, raspberries
Vegetables	Artichokes, collard greens, Brussels sprouts
Nuts and seeds	Almonds, sunflower seeds, chia seeds, flaxseeds

Table 2

FOODS RICH IN PREBIOTICS

Prebiotic Types	Examples
Oligofructose/Inulin	Onions, artichokes, banana, jicama, wild yam, chicory root
Beta-glucans	Oats, barley, wheat, rye, fungi
Pectins	Pears, apples, guavas, plums, citrus fruit, carrots, rose hips
Gums	Seeds, seaweed
Resistant starch	Bananas, lentils, peas, oats
Polyphenols	Berries, pomegranate, flaxseeds, sesame seeds, whole grains, chili peppers, oats, honey, apples, onions, dark chocolate, red cabbage, turmeric

Probiotics are live microorganisms that benefit your health. Many fermented foods contain high amounts of probiotics, but some processed fermented foods do not. When looking at foods traditionally full of probiotics, look for labels that say "live culture" or "active culture."

If you eat an anti-inflammatory, plant-based diet, food-based prebiotics and probiotics will be a part of your diet naturally. Supplements can be helpful in some situations, but they have their limitations. With probiotics, there are many things about the supplement to consider. What type of microbe is in the capsule? How much of the microbe does it contain? Will it still be alive and will it stay in your gut? Some people's microbiomes might be resistant to new microbes. We also don't have clear guidance on finding the best brands or types of probiotics. Probiotics come with few side effects, other than cost. It is reasonable to try a probiotic or other gut-supporting supplement under the supervision of your primary practitioner. Try to track your symptoms, and don't stay on a supplement that isn't providing you with some benefit. (For more, see Chapter 21 on natural products.)

Changing Your Diet to Help Your Gut Microbiome

We have only recently started to understand how truly bad for human health are the additives and ways we prepare processed foods. Many additives, flavorings, and fats are added to increase shelf life and make food look more appealing. But processed foods are associated with a rising risk of obesity, autoimmunity, and allergies in those who eat them. Processed foods change your microbiome.

The best thing you can do for your gut health is to eat a plant-based diet to decrease inflammation. Increasing your intake of fiber as well as prebiotic- and probiotic-containing foods will happen naturally when you shift your diet away from processed foods.

Studies have shown that changing your diet for only a few days can result in a major shift in your gut microbiome. That means you can improve some of your symptoms simply by changing your microbiome.

EXERCISE

MEDITATION: PREPARING TO REST AND DIGEST

You can do this meditation before eating, after eating, or both before and after eating.

Assume any comfortable position and close your eyes.

Rest your hands on your belly. Bring your attention to your breathing.

Bring your attention to your chest.

Your lungs, diaphragm, and stomach are here.

As you exhale, your diaphragm rises, and your stomach follows.

Your stomach is alive and ready to digest.

Bring your attention and your hands to your middle belly.

Your intestines live here.

Imagine your stomach muscles relaxing here, feeling warm and soft. As you draw your breath into your nose, allow it to fill your belly. Allow your belly to expand fully.

As you exhale, your abdomen and intestines become more relaxed.

Bring your attention to your lower belly, which holds your lower intestines.

As you breathe in, let the breath fill your lower belly and hold it there for a few seconds.

Slowly let the breath out. Allow your lower intestines to soften.

Feel the contact point of your pelvis and low back on the couch. This is the bottom of your abdominal cavity. These are the strong bones and muscles that support you.

With each breath, the connections between your gut and brain are signaling relaxation.

Your gut is resting, relaxed, and ready to digest.

Slowly come up to sitting and make your way to the table.

As you eat, take small bites, savor the flavor, and chew for just a few moments longer.

Return to the breath at any time.

CHAPTER 10

Sleep Disturbances and Insomnia

When I was diagnosed, I received a lot of steroids and a lot of other medications that really mess with your body. The insomnia started after the treatment, and it was just so incredibly frustrating because I was exhausted, I physically felt like I couldn't move my body.

I've been to multiple doctors and tried multiple medications and I think, out of all of my symptoms, insomnia is one of the most frustrating. There's fatigue, and then there's fatigue plus I haven't slept. I can't get any relief from it, I am just lying there in bed, and when you can't sleep, it's like every single ache and pain is worse.

At this point I'm on medicine for sleep. But some nights my brain is just going to do its thing no matter how hard you try to sedate it. It is really demoralizing, and it's sometimes downright depressing to just have this illness and have this fatigue and have all of these symptoms and just not be able to escape, no matter how much you want to, but also not have a way to refresh your body.

What You Will Learn in This Chapter:

- The physiology of sleep
- The risks of sleeping poorly for long periods of time
- The connection between sleep and long illness
- Signs and symptoms of common sleep disorders and when to see a specialist
- Science-backed strategies for tackling insomnia, including tools to help your brain learn to sleep again

Sleep regulates our mood, immune system, and memory. Without it, our bodies and minds cannot reclaim balance. Yet sleep is one of the first things that becomes disrupted when we get sick. Restful sleep, however, can supercharge recovery. In this chapter, we give you the knowledge and tools to optimize these essential hours. Your sleep time is anything but a snooze. During sleep, fascinating things happen in the body and mind. Let's dive in.

Sleep Stages and Cycles

Like the ocean, your sleep life is quiet on the surface but a rich world lies beneath. Each sleep stage serves an important function, and your body adjusts the amount of sleep you get in each stage nightly. You repeat this cycle throughout the night. On average, a sleep cycle is around ninety minutes. While your brain and mind are processing, your body is at work.

What Happens When You Get Good Sleep?

Experiences become memories, which are then stored in the brain.
Thinking and learning become easier.
Your mood and emotions become more balanced.
Your brain clears away waste and restores energy reserves.
Your hormones are regulated, including stress hormones.
Pain can improve.
Your metabolism speeds up.

What Happens When You Don't Sleep Enough?

Thinking and learning become harder.
Your emotional reactions are bigger, and you feel more anxiety, tension, and low mood.
Your brain holds on to more negative memories than positive ones, hardwiring you to feel negative about your world.
Sleep deprivation impairs your ability to understand other people's emotions; if you are chronically sleepy, you may have a harder time connecting meaningfully to other people.

Inflammation can increase.

Pain can worsen.

The immune system can weaken. People who get less than six hours of sleep have been shown to be four times more likely to catch a cold.

Your Circadian Rhythm

Your body has a unique internal clock called the *circadian rhythm*. A deep part of your brain responds to light and activity during your day and secretes the hormone melatonin. This hormone triggers your *sleep drive*.

Many of our recommendations involve supporting your circadian rhythm. Since light tells your brain when it is daytime and when it is nighttime, early morning natural light can help you get to sleep earlier. Similarly, evening light pushes your rhythm later. There are certain types of light that seem particularly damaging to sleep. The most common type: screens. The light that your phone or laptop screen emits disrupts the architecture of sleep and has been shown in studies to lead to increased daytime sleepiness. This is the science behind the general recommendation to put away your phone at least an hour before bed—and ideally earlier!

We also know that the circadian rhythm is closely linked to temperature. Because studies have shown that warm rooms increase alertness and decrease the amount of restful sleep, we recommend sleeping in a cool room.

Your sleep drive is your body's way of pushing you to sleep. You may have heard the expression "a wave of tired." This is a fairly typical description of the sleep drive at its strongest. It is most powerful in the evenings and weakest in the mornings. There are ways to strengthen your sleep drive, like staying awake during the day and reducing your caffeine intake.

Arousal is another factor that determines whether or not you sleep. Arousal is your level of alertness and attentiveness to the world around you. If your arousal is too strong, it will combat or overpower your sleep drive. People can feel more aroused when they are stressed, anxious, or traumatized.

What Is the Difference Between "Sleepy" and "Tired"?

It is important to distinguish "sleepy" from "tired." Your body is programmed to sleep and gives you the "I'm sleepy" message, which lets you know it is time to wind down. Once you can recognize this cue, it is easier to follow your body's internal rhythm. "Tired" is different. People can feel tired from exhaustion, fatigue, or illness. They may feel worn out, but it is different from "sleepy."

As you go about your day, try to reflect on these two feelings—sleepy and tired—and distinguish between the two. In people with long illness, this can be particularly challenging. Our patients often feel fatigue and tiredness throughout the day, and it can be hard to tell when this feeling shifts to sleepiness. Once you identify what sleepy feels like, you have begun to tap into your sleep driver. Trying to go to sleep when you are tired but not sleepy may be a challenge. Remember this distinction as we move through the rest of the chapter.

How Much Sleep Do You Need?

Most adults need seven to nine hours of sleep; small percentages of the population need less or more. In our experience, people with long illness do better when they get more sleep, not less. People who sleep too much or too little have a higher mortality risk. People who get less than six hours of sleep at night are also at an increased risk of developing dementia. This scary possibility is an important motivator to stay focused on improving sleep.

I'm very sensitive to not getting enough sleep, and I need much more sleep than a typical adult does. If I don't get enough rest I feel it cognitively very quickly. It can be very frustrating when that's going on and it feels like I just can't get the thoughts out. To survive, I really have to prioritize rest.

Sleep Problems

People with sleep problems can feel chronically depleted, wrung out, and hopeless. Here we review the most common medical sleep conditions, ways we diagnose them, and basic treatment. Insomnia and sleep apnea are the most common sleep disorders we see in long illness, so they have been given extra consideration in this chapter.

Sleep Apnea

Sleep apnea occurs when there is obstruction in breathing while you are sleeping. It can lead to less oxygen in the brain and be a strain on the heart. When left untreated, it can cause you to wake up often and make you incredibly sleepy. Sleep apnea is most common in people who are overweight but can be present in people of all shapes and sizes. Most people with sleep apnea have no idea that this is happening. They just feel exhausted during the day.

To diagnose this condition, a sleep study with oxygen monitoring is done either at home or in a sleep lab at a hospital. This can be ordered by a primary practitioner or a sleep specialist. Review the common symptoms of sleep apnea and talk to your practitioner if this sounds like something you are experiencing:

Apneas (times when your breathing pauses during sleep, usually witnessed by a person nearby)
Daytime sleepiness even after getting enough sleep
Dry mouth when you wake up
Headache when you wake up
Night awakenings
Snoring

Insomnia

Insomnia is a broad term. In medical terms, we diagnose it when someone has sleep difficulties three or more days of the week for more than three months. Sleep difficulties can be one or more of the following:

Difficulty falling asleep

Unwanted early-morning wake-ups

Waking up in the night with difficulty falling back to sleep

When diagnosing insomnia, we first rule out other sleep conditions, like sleep apnea. Another culprit is medications, including common medications for treating depression, asthma, and allergies. When discussing insomnia with your medical team, ask about the possibility of other sleep conditions and medications that could be worsening your sleep.

Sleep and Emotions

The hustle and bustle of the day can distract us from our feelings. Sleep pulls back the covers on what we have been avoiding. Often, when we address our emotional recovery, improvement in sleep follows.

Falling asleep is a process of letting go. Sometimes anxiety is too high to allow the mind to shut off. If your anxiety is high before bed, try exploring other tools for managing anxiety (Chapter 12).

Similarly, sleep disruption is one of the hallmarks of depression. It may be that treating your depression will help with sleep. It can't hurt to read more about depression (Chapter 11) and see if that possibility underlies some of your sleep difficulties.

Sleep makes us vulnerable. For some, it can feel less like falling asleep and more like falling off a cliff. To sleep we need to trust that we are safe enough to be able to rest. If trauma is a part of your story, sleep may not always feel safe. If this rings true for you, try incorporating an exercise like "Grounding with the Senses" before bed (Chapter 13). Working with a therapist around safety and sleep can also be a powerful way to optimize your sleep.

During sleepiness and sleep, we can no longer use our active defense mechanisms, like distraction. The guards we place at the gates of our anxieties go on break. For some people, especially those with fatigue or pain, bedtime can be a distressing experience, a time when they feel flooded with everything they have suppressed during the day. If this is happening to you, consider working with your health care team to manage your anxiety during the day.

Nightmares

Nightmares are common and often make sleep worse. About 5 percent of people experience one or more nightmares each week. Nightmares are associated with a diagnosis of post-traumatic stress disorder (see Chapter 13 on trauma). But nightmares are also more common in people with anxiety and depression. Our experience is that people who suffer from long illnesses have more nightmares. They are also common in people who have been hospitalized or undergone medical procedures.

Nightmares can be worsened by some sleep medications. Ask your practitioner if any of your medications could be giving you more nightmares.

Addressing nightmares is an important step in improving your sleep. An integrative approach to treating nightmares includes one or more of the following:

Hypnosis to use deep relaxation and guided suggestions to reduce nightmares

Medications that target reducing nightmare severity

Therapy to understand where the nightmares may be coming from and to reduce their intensity

If you have nightmares, scary and avoidant thoughts about sleep often pop up before bed. We recommend that you combat these thoughts by challenging them with thoughts that are more balanced. If fear of nightmares is keeping you awake, try this exercise to help you to feel safer.

EXERCISE

COGNITIVE BEHAVIORAL THERAPY

Try using the CBT skill of challenging negative thoughts about nightmares with alternative but realistic statements.

Distressing thought:

"I can't go to sleep because I will have a nightmare."

Alternative thought:

"I can fall asleep and know that I will be safe even if I have a nightmare."

Or:

"Nightmares are made of memories, they aren't really happening."

Or:

"I have been through so much and survived. Nightmares can't hurt me."

In your journal, write down some thoughts you can reach for to help you feel more grounded and secure before bed.

Restless Leg Syndrome

Some people have poor sleep because they have an irresistible urge to move their legs, often accompanied by an uncomfortable sensation. This is the description of a treatable condition called *restless leg syndrome* (RLS). We see this condition in people with long illness, especially those who are menstruating or have low iron levels (anemia) for other reasons. Once iron levels are restored, this distressing symptom can improve or even resolve completely. There are also other biomedicines that can be used to target this disruptive syndrome. An evaluation for RLS starts with a discussion with your primary practitioner.

Chronotypes and Disorders of Circadian Rhythm

Every person has their own unique sleep-wake cycle and rhythm. Most adults, around 60 percent, have an internal rhythm that aligns with societal patterns. They sleep at night and are awake during the day. However, approximately 40 percent of adults have a circadian rhythm that leans in the other direction. "Morning larks" are programmed to wake up extremely early, and "night owls" have a late rhythm. Your genetics probably dictate a large part of your chronotype, but your sleep rhythm is also influenced by environment, pain, mood, and exposure to light. When your chronotype affects your ability to function, we call it a disorder. We see many people with a long illness who have a *delayed sleep-wake phase* disorder. For these extreme "night owls," the disorder is highly disruptive to their life.

Early-morning light exposure shifts your sleep rhythm earlier, while light exposure later in the day shifts your sleep rhythm later. These shifts are ideally made with natural, bright light from the outdoors, but light therapy with a lamp in your home can also be effective. As we discuss in the mental health chapters, bright-light therapy can also treat most forms of depression.

If your chronotype is affecting your functioning, a sleep specialist or behavioral health practitioner can often help by using light therapy and natural products to gently shift your cycles to align your most productive hours more closely with daytime.

When to See a Sleep Specialist

Some rare sleep conditions and hard-to-treat sleep complaints are best evaluated by a sleep medicine specialist. Here are some reasons to talk to your primary care practitioner about a sleep medicine referral:

If your arms and legs move around at night and are keeping you awake

If you are acting out dreams, sleepwalking, or engaging in other strange behaviors at night

If you fall asleep when you don't want to, or in inappropriate places

If you have tried all of your primary practitioner's recommendations and are still not getting restful sleep

Treating Insomnia

The best-studied and most proven strategy to treat insomnia is cognitive behavior therapy for insomnia (CBTi). Much of the next section relies on

CBTi, as well as on the basic strategies we have learned through working with hundreds of people to help them sleep.

CBTi works better than our strongest sleep medications. Start by practicing the skills taught in this chapter. The best way to go deeper into CBTi is by asking your primary practitioner to refer you to a CBTi therapist or CBTi group. If this is unavailable in your area or inaccessible to you, check out our resources section for our favorite free CBTi app.

Treating insomnia is a three-step process: track, adjust, relax.

1. **Track:** When you track your sleep, you can see trends and identify your problem areas. Keeping a sleep diary can help you track your progress. It can also help you see trends over time and even identify potential triggers for poor sleep. Ideally, you want to make notes first thing in the morning, when the information is fresh in your mind. You can keep a sleep diary in your journal or on an app. Check out our resources section for our favorite CBTi and sleep diary apps.

Record the following information:
- The time you got into bed
- How long it took you to fall asleep
- The time when you fell asleep
- The time and duration of any awakenings
- The time you woke up
- The quality of your sleep
- Any naps you took during the day

Additional information:
- How much caffeine you consumed
- Your pain level
- Your stress level

2. **Adjust:** The trends you see when you track your sleep can help you make targeted changes.

If you have trouble falling asleep:

- Go to sleep *only* when sleepy. Wait until you feel your sleep drive kick in before you get in bed.
- Put away devices that wake up your brain:
  o Put down your electronics and screens at least an hour before bed.
  o Consider putting your phone out of reach of the bed.
  o Try using a digital clock rather than looking at your phone overnight. Turn the clock around so you don't automatically look at it during a wake-up.
- Train your brain to expect sleep:
  o Go to bed at the same time each night.
  o Wake up at the same time each morning.
  o Make your bed a place for no activities except sleep and sexual intimacy.
- Prepare your "sleep sanctuary": Prepare your sleep space so it is cool, dark, and quiet. (Purchase stick-on blackout shades and a sound machine if you haven't done so already.) Any light in the room can block your sleep drive.
- Put aside worrying: Schedule a twenty-minute "worry period" during the day. Try completing the "Drifting Thoughts" exercise provided here. Offload worry from your mind before bed.
- Exercise: Exercise during the day can help with sleep at night, so start an exercise regimen by reading Chapter 19. Be careful with the timing of exercise. Avoid exercise right before bed, as the endorphins released can override your sleep drive.
- Avoid caffeine: Caffeine stays active in your system for many hours after your last cup, so avoid having it after lunch and at least five hours before bedtime.
- Avoid naps: Naps lasting more than fifteen to twenty minutes can reduce your sleep drive. Try to nap only if you can't function without one, and keep it short whenever possible.

- Relax: Practice mindfulness meditation. Try the "Drifting Thoughts" exercise or any other meditation you have enjoyed from another chapter.
- Avoid large meals late in the day: Try not to eat in the two to four hours before going to bed and avoid foods that can upset your stomach.

If you experience multiple awakenings:
- Reduce your fluid intake after dinner.
- Don't look at the clock or at a screen upon awakening. In fact, try not to watch the clock at all. Just go back to sleep when you feel sleepy.
- Consider a weighted blanket.
- If you are awake and don't easily get back to sleep, get out of bed and do something relaxing.

If the quality of your sleep is poor:
- Avoid alcohol: Alcohol can be sedating and help people fall asleep, but the quality of sleep when alcohol is in your system is impaired. Alcohol weakens your body's natural sleep rhythms and can lead to drowsiness during the day, even if you get enough hours of sleep at night.
- Put down your phone before bed.
- Increase exercise during the day.
- Increase exposure to natural light earlier in the day.
- Discuss with your primary care practitioner whether any of your medications could be affecting your sleep.
- Talk with your health care team about whether another sleep condition is contributing to your poor sleep and whether you need a referral to a sleep specialist.

3. **Relax:** Your sleep needs to be stronger than your level of arousal or alertness in order to push you into sleep. You can modify your level of arousal by optimizing relaxation. There are many different ways to relax:

Incorporate movement into your day.

Address your anxiety during the day, so that it doesn't accumulate and amplify before bed.

Develop a relaxing night ritual. The exercise provided here will help you develop a personalized plan.

Incorporate self-massage.

Use mindfulness to tune into a more relaxing wavelength.

EXERCISE

MINDFULNESS: "DRIFTING THOUGHTS"

You can use this mindfulness exercise, which is inspired by CBT, to develop a new relationship with your thinking. It can be especially helpful around sleep.

Have you ever lain on the ground and watched clouds go by overhead? They move and shift and float out of view. Some look like scary shapes at first, but then they shift and change. We don't try to grab the clouds or change them. We don't give them names. We allow them to pass until they are out of view.

In this exercise, you will view your thoughts as though they are clouds simply passing by. Try this exercise for a few minutes as part of your evening relaxation routine. Read the instructions here or record yourself reading them and play back the recording:

Set a five-minute timer. Lie down on your back in a quiet space. Close your eyes. Try to visualize clouds overhead. Breathe deeply and relax. As a thought comes into your mind, place it on a cloud. Watch that cloud move and drift away. There is no need to examine the cloud, take the thought down off the cloud, or linger. Let the thought drift out of view. You are safe and whole. Your thoughts can drift past.

As thoughts move into your mind, place them one by one on a cloud. Allow them to drift away. Keep breathing. Keep noticing your thoughts. Stay with your breath.

Consider using some of the meditations in other parts of this book and incorporating them into your bedtime routine. We think that the progressive muscle relaxation (page 178) and safe space (page 186) meditations are particularly relaxing and useful before bed.

EXERCISE

RELAX BEFORE BED

Knowing what is relaxing for your mind and body can help you tailor your bedtime routine and find relaxing practices to employ if you wake up at night. Here is a list of relaxing activities that don't involve screens, which we know can activate parts of the brain that fight sleep. Are any of these practices relaxing for you?

Reading	Hot beverage	Heating pad	Gentle stretching	Cold beverage
Shower	Self-massage	Mantras	Making the bed	Journaling
Breathing	Weighted blanket	Prayer	Hair and nail care	Ice pack
Holding a soothing object	Listening to a podcast	Listening to music	Cuddling a pet	Bath

What relaxing practices can you include in your nighttime routine?

Pain and Sleep

Pain can disrupt sleep, either by making it hard to fall asleep or by waking you up in the night. We recommend making a pain care plan that addresses disruption from pain overnight as much as possible. Strategies for relieving pain at night include self-massage, heat or ice, and evening-administered medications. Refer to Chapter 4 for more on addressing pain.

Medications and Natural Products

The goal with any sleep medication is to use it for only a short time while you address the underlying reasons for your poor sleep. Even with short-term use, most sedating sleep medications affect the quality of sleep and disrupt the natural cycles and phases of sleep. When this happens, sleep may not be as replenishing. Many of our most commonly used sleep medications, like Benadryl and Ambien, are associated with an increased risk of dementia and falls if used over the long term. If you do need more support around sleep, we recommend using non-habit-forming medications whenever possible.

Natural products are also frequently used for insomnia. The most commonly used is melatonin, which supplements a hormone already made by your body and is low-risk and effective when taken at least one hour before bedtime. Other common natural products used for sleep are valerian root, lemon balm, tryptophan, GABA, glycine, chamomile, oral lavender, and magnesium. Talk with your health care team about whether a natural sleep product would be right for you and, as always, make sure there are no contraindications with any medications you are taking.

What to Do When You're Frustrated and Worried and Lying Awake

Very few things are as frustrating as being awake when you want to be asleep. This frustration is normal, but it fuels the insomnia, making it worse. Here are two evidence-based strategies for reducing the worry associated with getting to sleep.

EXERCISE

SCHEDULE A "WORRY" TIME

Pick a twenty-minute time slot during the day when you will allow your mind to worry. Make sure to keep this worry time from running over—limit it to thirty minutes max. This scheduled worry time during the day shows your mind that you are addressing its concerns and can reduce worry that might otherwise arise when you're trying to go to sleep.

EXERCISE

PRE-SLEEP TO-DO LISTS

We've all woken up thinking about things we need to do. One study looked at whether writing a to-do list before bed could help us avoid this interruption to our sleep. And it did. People who wrote out specific lists of things they needed to do the next day or week got to sleep faster and woke up less often.

Try writing out a to-do list thirty minutes before bed. We recommend including things you can worry about later. Complete this list prior to your wind-down period. Then put it aside and relax. You can add things as basic as getting pet food or worrying about bills another day.

Even with these tools in hand, you can have bad nights. Insomnia often has an ebb and flow, and it can take time for your brain to learn how to sleep in a new way. So what can you do at night when worry and frustration arise? Rather than getting onto the roller coaster of worry, try practicing mindfulness. Just notice the roller coaster, but don't go for a ride on it. We like using the above mindfulness exercise to help with relaxation and to cultivate space between our thoughts and experiences.

Journaling

Write down three new facts you learned about your sleep.

Make a list of some of the practices in this chapter that resonated with you. Which one are you prepared to try this week? How do you think it will change your sleep?

How Can You Continue to Improve Your Sleep?

If sleep is still a struggle for you, focus on understanding what helps your mind know that it is appropriate to fall asleep. Maybe you need to focus on lowering your overall anxiety levels, or explore trauma treatment, or leave your phone in another room. You could also try venturing into other healing modalities that can help with sleep, like self-massage (page 108), energy work, or acupuncture.

Struggling with insomnia can powerfully reinforce it. After we take small actions, the results are out of our control, and so acceptance becomes a part of treatment. This may be where you are now, but it's unlikely that you'll be here forever.

Take a small action, then turn over the results. Accept your current struggle (insomnia), and ask for help when you need it. If you aim for progress, not perfection, sleep is likely to follow.

PART III

MENTAL HEALTH

Experiences with illness are scary and painful. Anxiety, depression, insomnia—these are natural responses to problems like inflammation, pain, and brain fog, and your mind is sounding the alarm. Even though feelings come factory-installed in every human, long illness can give you the message that your feelings are wrong. Some of the biological changes and genetic differences associated with long illnesses can make a person more vulnerable to mental health problems. Long illness impacts the nervous system and increases inflammation, which changes emotional networks in the brain. These impacts can overload your emotional system and cause myriad mental health problems, including anxiety and depression. Adding in past (or present) trauma and the stress of relationships, current events, and the many roadblocks in life can make it all too much to bear. In a long illness you've got a perfect storm of mental health risk that, if left unaddressed, could spiral into a mental health crisis.

Your brain and body are intimately connected. Leaving psychological distress untreated increases inflammation. Ignoring or brushing aside your emotional suffering can often worsen a long illness.

We are here to normalize the emotional battles that arise out of long illness and give you resources and tools to cope and restore your center. In the following chapters we have chosen to focus on the three common struggles in long illness: depression, anxiety, and trauma. We cover them in separate chapters simply for the sake of organization; for most people these conditions are intertwined. That said, there are many issues related to mental health that are equally deserving of time, attention, and treatment but that we do not have room to discuss. We have addressed some of these diagnoses in the resources section, and we believe that many of the concepts introduced here can be applied to a broad range of mental health issues. Make sure to connect with your health care team about any mental health concerns you have that are not addressed in this book.

One of our recommendations that you will see throughout these chapters, therapy, comes in many forms. Some therapy uses tools that are easy to share in this book, like exercises and images. Others, like "talk" therapy (psychodynamic therapy), are powerful and effective but don't lend themselves to written exercises. The type of therapy you choose is probably less important than finding a therapist you connect with and feel is helpful.

Your relationship with your therapist is as important as the treatment itself. Ideally, you and your therapist have a shared understanding of your struggles and the pathway forward. If possible, it can be useful to ask a screening question before booking a visit with a therapist:

"Have you worked with anyone before with an illness like mine? If not, are you open to learning more?"

In many areas of the country, mental health practitioners are hard to access. It may be your primary care practitioner who provides your mental health care. Many of these practitioners are excellent at managing common psychological complaints, but if you're still suffering, ask your practitioner for a referral to a specialist. You can also use our resources section to gather ideas for getting psychological care.

Nobody wants to feel depressed, anxious, or chronically traumatized. But exploring those bad feelings as a focus of treatment can be terrifying.

Getting treatment for your mental health often involves moving toward precisely the feeling you have been trying to avoid. We know this feels scary. Hopelessness can also be a barrier to treatment ("I've done this before and it never helped"). But we have seen people finally find mental health solutions that help them after years of suffering. It can be hard to push forward, but you deserve more.

We acknowledge that everyone reading this will approach these chapters with varying experiences. Whatever you bring with you, we hope there is something for you here.

CHAPTER 11

Depression

I had just ended a job. I was in therapy. I was trying a bunch of different supplements, and having a hard time sleeping. I was having more pain. And this depression came over me like it never had before. Like I was stuck at the bottom of the pool. Nothing felt right. I wanted to sleep all day. It felt like nothing was going to be okay. I was crying at the drop of a hat. I didn't know how I would get through it.

I ended up learning that my sleep medicine was making my depression worse, as well as one of my supplements. I stopped both of those, and it got a little better. I didn't want to sleep all day. But I still wasn't out yet. It was a combination of a lot of things that got me back. I didn't want to do medications, but maybe I should have. I'm okay today, my pain is less, I don't have those terrifying thoughts, and I'm back to talking about things in therapy. I don't want to experience that again.

What You Will Learn in This Chapter:

- How long illness can both cause and worsen depression
- How treating depression can improve long illness
- The many treatment options for depression
- Exercises and journaling to allow you to reflect on the impact of depression on your life

Depression is one of the most common problems that people with long illness face.

Depression is lonely. It's hard to imagine that someone else can understand how it feels. If you feel this way, it is time to talk to your health care team. Primary care practitioners and mental health practitioners are trained in helping with these feelings.

We are here to help you too.

Once depression settles in your mind, it can be hard to change on your own. Even when part of you wants to get well, that part often gets over-powered. The depressed brain is afraid of change and too stuck to try new things. For some people, depression runs so deep that they think about ending their life. Suicidal thoughts are common and serious among people who are depressed, especially those with a long illness, who have a hard time envisioning a future that feels different.

If you are having suicidal thoughts, or thoughts of wishing you didn't exist, you need more help. Pick someone close to you—a friend, a family member, a health care worker—and tell them. If you feel like you could hurt yourself, call the 988 Suicide & Crisis Lifeline at 988, or head to the emergency room NOW. You are in a life-or-death situation, so don't wait.

The depressed brain says things won't get better, and it often feels like too much to bear. But depression can get better. We know because we see it happening every day.

> *I had never really had depression before I got sick. It took me a long time to recognize. My gut was really messed up, I was fatigued, it is depressing to be sick, it's depressing to accept current circumstances when they change. I had to grieve the life I had previously. For me, depression was a stage of grief. I had to grieve for my healthy, able-bodied life. Depression was a stage of that. It was more complicated than that too. My gut health, my fatigue, my body was impacting my depression as well.*

Understanding Your Depression

We are still discovering all the roots of depression. What is clear is that depression is not a one-size-fits-all illness. Your experience of depression probably feels different than another person's. Depression is a label that covers many distinct problems that have several symptoms in common.

While you read, pay attention to the explanations that relate to *your* depression. This chapter is designed to help you put together the puzzle pieces of your unique experience.

Biological explanations for depression:

- **Low levels of neurotransmitters:** Neurotransmitters are the messaging chemicals of the brain. Three neurotransmitters—serotonin, dopamine, and norepinephrine—balance your mood. In long illness, levels of these neurotransmitters can be depleted.
- **Disruption in brain circuits:** Long illness affects important brain networks called *circuits*, which regulate mood and emotions. And because the brain is interconnected, many other brain functions essential for helping you get through your days can be dulled as well.
- **Secondary depression:** Some depression is caused by vitamin deficiencies, hormone changes, infections, or medication side effects. This is why seeing a medical practitioner to screen for secondary causes is so important.
- **Genetic factors:** Are there other people in your family who have been depressed? Such genetic vulnerabilities may be more prevalent in people with long illness.
- **Inflammation and pain:** Inflammation and pain can also affect your mood and cause depression.

Psychological explanations for depression:

- Anger expressed toward yourself
- Walled-off or repressed emotions
- Parental attachment wounds; caregivers who were not able to care for emotional needs or who responded to needs in mean or confusing ways
- Invalidation and identity disturbance
- Loss and grief

- Trauma and abuse
- Unsupportive or abusive relationships
- Societal messages; discrimination; shame; and judgment

Philosophical and spiritual explanations for depression:
- Loss of "vital" energy
- Lack of purpose
- Spiritual struggles

Journaling

WHERE DOES MY DEPRESSION COME FROM?

Now that you have identified the unique roots of your depression, use your journal to explore further. This can be helpful when you are choosing from among the treatments we discuss next. Write down the following categories and add your thoughts.

	Examples
Biological	Genetics: Mom and brother both have depression too Circuits: My depression also makes me have problems with memory, so it makes sense that my depression is connected to other parts of my brain
Psychological	Anger toward self Low self-esteem Loss/grief: Dad died last year
Philosophical/Spiritual	Being in nature feels spiritual to me Connecting with nature makes me feel better Going to mosque makes me feel calm

Treating Your Depression

We've broken this down into two steps.

Step 1: Get connected. Your primary care practitioner should be able to refer you to a mental health practitioner if you need more support. There are two big distinctions in mental health care:

Medical practitioners: Primary care practitioners, psychiatrists, nurse-practitioners, and physician's assistants can prescribe medications to treat your depression and other symptoms it can cause, and they sometimes offer psychotherapy. They are trained to evaluate for medical problems masquerading as mental health problems.

Nonmedical psychotherapists: There are many different training programs for therapists. Therapists with a master's degree in social work (MSW), a master's in family therapy (MFT), or a doctorate (PhD), as well as licensed clinical therapists and others, can provide talk therapy and support those working through their depression. They cannot prescribe medications.

Step 2: Choose a treatment.

Psychotherapy (talk therapy): There is excellent evidence for the treatment of depression with psychotherapy. Psychotherapy can be done in a structured way, such as in cognitive behavioral therapy, which focuses on building skills and understanding of behavior, thoughts, and emotions. Other types of psychotherapy use psychological understanding to guide the client in a more open-ended format.

Medications: Some people are hesitant about taking a pill that might change how they think or feel. But these medications can often be life-changing in long illness, because the most common antidepressant medications also have anti-inflammatory properties. Your practitioner can even choose one that doubles as a pain reliever, or one that can also reduce nausea, increase your appetite, sharpen your focus, or improve your sleep. And people can feel a lot better once inflammation is reduced, pain is reduced, and brain chemicals are more balanced.

Finding the right treatment for your depression may take some time and adjustments. If you are medication-sensitive, talk to your mental health or primary practitioner about customized dosing (including liquid formulations) so that you can take the medication at your own pace. There are several different types of antidepressants. If your current medication isn't working, there may be another antidepressant that does work for you.

Supplements: Several natural products are excellent in the treatment of depression, either alone or in combination with biomedicines. The natural products we use most often in treating depression are St. John's wort, saffron, L-methylfolate, 5-hydroxytryptophan (5HTP), acetyl-L-carnitine, omega-3 fatty acids, S-Adenosyl methionine (SAMe), N-acetylcysteine, magnesium, vitamin D, probiotics, oral lavender (Silexan), adaptogens, and turmeric. Always talk to your practitioner before starting a supplement; you'll want to make sure that it's right for you and your condition, and that there are no contraindications with any other medications you're taking. Refer to Chapter 21 for a guide to supplements and natural products.

Lifestyle changes: When you are depressed—and especially if you have chronic pain and fatigue—the last thing you may feel like doing is exercising or paying attention to how you eat. We want to recognize and honor these complicated feelings. As with every other suggestion in this book, we encourage you to take small steps.

Exercise: Studies have shown us that exercise can act as an antidepressant. Refer to Chapter 19 to explore starting a movement routine, even if you live with pain and fatigue.

Diet: A healthy diet can improve depression. Skip to Chapter 17 to learn more. Consider keeping a food diary to track not only what you eat but your moods and feelings at the time.

Increased social support: Reaching out to social networks and making new friends can help with depression. Support groups are an excellent way to build social support with people who are also living with depression. Look at our resources section for more information on support groups.

Integrative medicine modalities: These are four evidence-based treatments that we frequently recommend to anyone with long illness and depression.

1. **Light therapy:** We initially used light therapy only for those with seasonal affective disorder (a worsening mood in the darker months), but now we know that light therapy can be effective in treating many forms of depression. You can purchase a light therapy lamp or bulb inexpensively online. When you are purchasing a light, look for a brightness of at least 10,000 lux with a UV filter to protect your skin and eyes.

2. **Acupuncture:** In studies, people with depression who paired acupuncture with medications did better than people who took medications alone. Check out Chapter 20 on traditional medicine for a deeper explanation of acupuncture.

3. **Yoga:** We have seen excellent results in our practice using yoga to help with recovery from depression, and studies have confirmed yoga's effectiveness. In Chapter 19 on exercise, we discuss yoga in depth.

4. **Mindfulness/meditation:** Start with moving meditations or guided visualizations if being too still feels uncomfortable to you. Yoga is a form of meditation, so if you try a sequence for depression, you will be hitting three of our suggestions here (exercise, yoga, meditation) at once!

Brain stimulation therapies: When other forms of treatment don't work, some people with depression turn to procedures in which specialized psychiatrists use electrodes or magnets to stimulate the brain. Here are the two most common treatments:

1. **Transcranial magnetic stimulation (TMS):** TMS uses magnets to create electrical changes in areas of the brain that control mood and perceive pain.
2. **Electroconvulsive therapy (ECT):** ECT is a treatment for people who have severe depression that has not responded to other types of treatment. There are many myths and outdated ideas about ECT, but rest assured that it is safe—and it has been proven effective for treatment-resistant depression.

> **Emerging treatments:** Ketamine, a medication that was once used only for pain management, is being used in psychiatry to boost mood. It has a "dissociative" effect, which means that you can feel separated from your mind or body during the treatment.
>
> **Psychedelic treatments:** Psilocybin (magic mushrooms) and MDMA (ecstasy) are being studied for their potential to treat depression and post-traumatic stress disorder (PTSD). Initial studies have been promising. They are not currently available in clinical practice, but research is ongoing. See our resources section for a link to a clinical trials database.

Talk to your practitioner about these treatments if you have tried many of the other options and have found no relief.

Journaling

What is your philosophy around treating depression? What has worked for you? What hasn't? Is there anything you want to explore more? Are you open to revisiting things that might not have worked in the past?

Core Beliefs

We all carry core beliefs about ourselves that build our self-esteem. Holding many negative core beliefs can contribute to depression. And getting "stuck" in untreated depression worsens long illness.

Here are examples of negative common core beliefs:

I am broken.
I will feel bad forever.
I am not good enough.
I am defective.
I am unlovable.
I am a bad person.
Other people can't be trusted.
I cannot ask for help.
I cannot handle things.
I am weak.
People I love leave me.

You may identify with one or several of these negative core beliefs. Again, these are common beliefs to hold.

Journaling

CHALLENGING CORE BELIEFS

In most cases, our negative core beliefs are reflections of being stuck in memories of how we were treated, not a reflection of who we are. If you carry painful core beliefs about yourself and want to see if those can shift, try exploring this further with us. But if focusing on negative core beliefs doesn't feel good and you feel that it wouldn't help your recovery right now, that's okay. If you start to do this work and find that it is activating or triggering, feel free to put it down. If you have a trusted person in your life with whom you feel safe discussing this, like a therapist, you could resume with that person's support.

Core beliefs attract the things that confirm that they are true and repel the contradictory evidence. This means that negative core beliefs have you holding on to the negatives and not the positives. Here is an example:

"I Am Defective"	
Why I Think This Is True	Why This Is Not True
I have been sick for so long I have tried lots of things and nothing helps I am more sensitive than other people My trauma means I am never okay	I have many good days Acupuncture has helped, and so have a few other things I am intuitive and smart, and this is a gift I have good insight about my body My illness does not rob me of my value

In your journal, write out up to three of your core beliefs. On one side of the page, write down what supports the belief. On the other side, write down what argues against it.

CHAPTER 12

Anxiety and Stinking Thinking

Sometimes I just get stuck in these terrible thoughts, and I can't get out. Every-thing feels like it is going wrong and I can't see past this moment. With every bad thought, my body hurts more and my mind races. In those moments, the experience feels almost infinite. While I know it always ends, my body won't let me remember in the moment. I can completely go from bumping my knee in the grocery store to sobbing in my car moments later, having leapt to the conclusion that no one will ever love me because I am sick.

Therapy has really helped give me a list of things I can do when I am going down the spiral. I do things like text friends, challenge my thoughts, and distract myself. Later I write down and reflect on these events and talk about them with my therapist. It's not perfect, but it made a big difference.

What You Will Learn in This Chapter:

- The neuroscience of anxiety and its many layers in the brain and body
- Treatment options for addressing anxiety in long illness
- Skills for acknowledging and releasing body-based emotions
- Tools you can practice to move toward your values

Most of us have felt anxious. Your thoughts race, your muscles tense, and your heart speeds up. There is a tightness in your chest. A buzz-ing energy fills your body, like a can of soda that has been shaken and not opened. These feelings often pass. But when they don't, your system can go into overdrive and stop you from living the life you want.

Anxiety may manifest in the body, or it could be generated as a response to the body. This is one of the reasons why heightened anxiety is common in long illnesses. When the body struggles, so does the mind.

Anxiety is naturally generated in response to common symptoms in long illness, like pain, shortness of breath, or indigestion. But this signal can get overamplified. A little bit of anxiety can be helpful, but chronic anxiety increases inflammation, depletes neurotransmitters, and changes networks in the brain. When these symptoms aren't going away overnight, the brain needs to recalibrate. This often doesn't happen without doing some form of psychological work.

Repeated experiences in our health care system of invalidation and helplessness can also worsen anxiety. Anxiety flares can worsen symptoms. And symptom flares can worsen anxiety. This is why addressing anxiety is so essential for those with a long illness.

Relieving anxiety is often a process of small improvements before relief is felt, but there are some evidence-informed strategies that do eventually reduce anxiety: journaling, CBT, and mindfulness. Other approaches are newer, like exercises inspired by acceptance and commitment therapy (ACT) and somatic work.

You can also lean on your health care team. If your anxiety prevents you from living your life to the fullest, it's time to talk to your primary care practitioner or a skilled mental health practitioner. Anxiety and depression use the same connections (aka circuits) and chemicals in the brain, so many of the same treatments for depression are used to treat anxiety.

Anxiety and Your Nervous System

Anxiety is behind the wheel of the race car that is your fight-or-flight sympathetic nervous system. And when fight-or-flight is out of balance, anxiety is high. There is a feedback loop: a heightened sympathetic nervous system increases anxiety, and anxiety revs the engine of the sympathetic nervous system. It is a vicious cycle.

We emphasize mindfulness again because it strengthens your calming rest-and-digest parasympathetic nervous system. It can balance and reduce anxiety when practiced consistently. (Make sure to dive into the foundational tools section of Chapter 1 for other ways to rebalance your system.)

Your Default Mode Network

There are times when anxiety will be high for a period of time, then it passes. A good example is final exams. Your anxiety fuels your studying, and then you can relax. But for many people with a long illness, relaxation never comes.

To understand this type of anxiety, we look to neuroscience. Your brain is like a computer. It has a screensaver mode, which is a part of your brain superhighway system called the *default mode network*. It is active when you are no longer distracted by the external world. In people with depression and anxiety, this network looks different.

The problem for many people is that their screensaver is filled with anxieties, from worries about the future or the past to fears about their health and painful core beliefs about themselves. When their brains should be

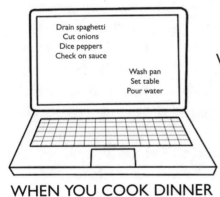

Drain spaghetti
Cut onions
Dice peppers
Check on sauce

Wash pan
Set table
Pour water

WHEN YOU COOK DINNER

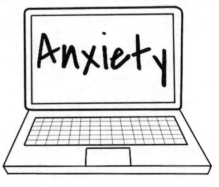

WHEN YOUR MIND WANDERS

Anxiety

"shutting off" and relaxing, these messages only get louder. Many people experience this part of their brain kicking in right before sleep as they are trying to rest. Anxiety is their default mode.

It can be helpful to think about this dimension of anxiety in your own brain. What is on the screensaver of your brain's computer? Most of the time this screensaver kicks in without you knowing it. Pause and take a moment to understand what is in the background of your mind. Just noticing it is a helpful first step to shifting its contents.

Journaling

What are the thoughts and feelings that pop up when you aren't in the middle of a task or distracted?

Your Relationship to Anxiety

Many people have a conflicted relationship with their anxiety. They might feel that it pushes them to get work done, to call family, to exercise. It keeps them going, even when they are tired.

Anxiety is a normal part of being a human. However, people often misinterpret how much their anxiety is doing for them. Most of the time it generates more exhaustion than productivity. In a long illness, your anxiety might feel like it is an important alarm system to let you know how your body is doing. Anxiety might be what eventually motivates you to attend appointments or engage in self-care. Anxiety might also be a way of avoiding more painful underlying feelings, like illness-related grief. In most cases, your mind is trying to protect you by generating anxiety, but it's also depleting you.

Many people hate their anxiety, but the prospect of letting go of worrying leaves them feeling even more uncomfortable. Sometimes we hold on to anxiety because it's our primary way of coping. Anxiety can feel like control. Anxiety may also be covering up deeper feelings under the surface, like grief and sadness. Or a deep sense of being unsafe or unseen. These feelings are guarded by anxiety, which prevents them from being processed and expressed. And the longer those feelings go undigested, the worse the anxiety may get.

It can be useful to understand why your anxiety is being generated so strongly, and what is holding you back from releasing it, even if understanding comes only a little bit at a time. Getting *curious* about your anxiety and examining it can help you understand its function, hopefully reduce its intensity, and be a step toward acceptance.

Journaling

Who would you be without anxiety? How different would your day be? What is your relationship to anxiety?

What does your anxiety do *for* you? Write about a time when your anxiety helped you accomplish something.

Write about a time when your anxiety prevented you from accomplishing a goal or doing something you enjoy. How is your anxiety working against you?

Psychotherapy

Some anxiety can be addressed with psychotherapy alone. Again, there isn't just one type of therapy that works best or is supported by the best evidence. We see from the medical literature that it is the quality of the attachment to the therapist that makes all of the difference. If you trust your therapist and think they are helping you, you are doing the right type of therapy.

Medications

The medications for treating anxiety that are supported by the best evidence are antidepressants, most probably because they treat the symptoms underlying anxiety. There are also medications that directly target anxiety, without addressing mood. Unfortunately, some of these are habit-forming and have significant risks; benzodiazepines, for example, are linked to memory problems and can increase the risk of falls. People can develop a tolerance for these medications and require escalating doses to control their symptoms. There are also non-habit-forming medications that can be taken as needed for anxiety, although these seem to work best when the roots of the anxiety are also addressed with either antidepressant medications or psychotherapy. Several natural products can be used to treat anxiety, including oral lavender (Silexan), ginkgo, passionflower, and magnesium. All medications work best when coupled with therapy.

Experiential Avoidance

We often try hard to run away from anxiety. It is natural to want to protect ourselves. For example, if you get anxious around groups of people, you might choose to stay home even though you'll miss out on spending time with loved ones. This is called *experiential avoidance*, and it can negatively impact your life. When we try to avoid anxiety, we often make decisions that move us *away* from the people, experiences, and values that are important to us. In long illness, avoidance can look like procrastinating, delaying health maintenance, isolating, or coping in ways that are comforting but not health-promoting. When we run from our anxiety, it gets bigger and our world gets smaller.

The opposite of experiential avoidance is acceptance, which does not mean rolling over or giving up. Acceptance is allowing yourself to feel anxiety instead of avoiding it. When you make room for your anxiety, you give yourself permission to make choices that move you *toward* being the person you want to be, even when those choices are frightening.

The concept of experiential avoidance comes from a school of therapy called acceptance and commitment therapy. ACT hinges on the idea that aligning with your values and moving toward them, even when it means moving toward some anxiety, can lead to greater mental flexibility and a more meaningful life. Check out our resources section for ways to learn more ACT concepts.

EXERCISE

CHOICES

We all can make a choice between avoidance and acceptance. When we make choices in line with our values, or with vitality as a whole, we are likely to build greater satisfaction into our lives. This exercise is inspired by acceptance and commitment therapy.

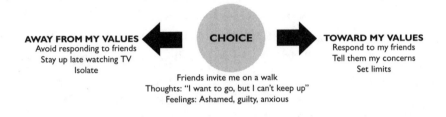

AWAY FROM MY VALUES
Avoid responding to friends
Stay up late watching TV
Isolate

CHOICE

TOWARD MY VALUES
Respond to my friends
Tell them my concerns
Set limits

Friends invite me on a walk
Thoughts: "I want to go, but I can't keep up"
Feelings: Ashamed, guilty, anxious

In the example exercise shown here is a person who values building community. Her friends invite her to go for a walk, but she fears that she will not be able to keep up, or that her fatigue will be too overwhelming. She has a choice to make: she can move away from her values, which may temporarily provide relief but will not lead to satisfaction or a long-term reduction in her anxiety. This choice would be experiential avoidance. Or she can move toward her values, accepting that this choice probably means sitting with some anxiety as well. But moving toward her values will reduce her anxiety in the long run. The rightward arrow allows her to continue to pursue community while also responding to her friends and setting appropriate limits on the walk.

A choice in line with her values moves this person toward things that make her anxious, like communicating with friends and setting limits. You may also experience more short-term anxiety when you make choices in line with your values, but doing so can lower your anxiety over the long run. Try thinking about the choices in your life right now. What pulls you away from your values? What pulls you toward them? Can you cultivate some willingness to reflect on your choices? Try this the next time you are facing a challenging situation.

MEDITATION: UNLOCKING BODY FEELINGS

Close your eyes. Allow your mind to focus on each individual area of your body, from your toes to the top of your head. Ask, "What experiences has this body part been through? What emotions are here?"

Take three deep breaths.

Scan your body, starting with your feet and rising to your head. Try to remain open to any feelings or experiences held in the body. Allow yourself to feel whatever may arise. If at any point it starts to feel too intense, take a break. Keep breathing. Use each breath as a tool for clearing away anything you no longer want to hold within.

Bring your awareness to your feet. Breathe deeply and connect the rest of your body with your feet. People think about their feet in different ways. For some, their feet carry them long distances, while others experience pain in their feet. Are you carrying any emotions in your feet? Are any experiences held there? With the next breath, try to release with the exhale anything you don't want to hold on to.

Bring your awareness to your legs. Legs bear tremendous responsibility. Today they may feel strong, weak, or even painful. Are there feelings that come up when you shift your attention to your legs? Are any experiences held there? With the next breath, try to release with the exhale anything you don't want to hold on to.

Bring your attention to your hips and abdomen. Pause here. Breathe deeply. Notice any feelings that arise. These areas can be tender, vulnerable, and filled with memories that are both conscious and unconscious. Are there memories still residing in your hips and abdomen? On your next breath, allow anything ready to be released to ride the wave of your next exhale.

Bring your attention to your chest. Feel it rise and fall. Notice if anything comes up for you when you hold your attention here. Are there memories or emotions residing in your chest? On your next breath, allow anything ready to release to ride the wave of your next exhale.

Bring your attention to your neck, the space of your voice, your self-expression. Notice if anything comes up for you when you hold your attention here. Are there memories or emotions residing in your neck? On your next breath, allow anything ready to release to ride the wave of your next exhale.

Bring your attention to your arms. Breathe deeply, experiencing your arms and hands fully. Notice if anything comes up for you when you hold your attention here. Do memories or emotions reside in your arms? On your next breath, allow anything ready to release to ride the wave of your next exhale.

Bring your attention to your face and head. Your brain has processed all of your experiences, and your face has expressed your emotions. Breathe deeply, experiencing your face and head fully. Notice if anything comes up for you when you hold your attention here. Are there memories or emotions residing in your head or in your face? On your next breath, allow anything ready to release to ride the wave of your next exhale.

Give yourself time to linger in any area where more information may be available. Breathe deeply, slowly, and continuously. Use the information gathered during this meditation to expand on your understanding in the next exercise.

Stinking Thinking

In a long illness, you want to understand your thinking as much as possible, and how it may be impacting your illness. You can start by recognizing that anxiety is often generated out of a state of fear, shame, or depression. Automatic negative thoughts, or "stinking" thoughts, usually go with it. These thoughts often play on loop, plaguing you and revving up your anxiety. The more self-insulting and catastrophic your thinking gets, the worse the anxiety becomes.

Automatic negative thoughts are rarely a reflection of the whole truth. They are mostly black-and-white thinking, lacking any perspective that incorporates shades of gray. Once you gain some insight and perspective on these thoughts, you can lessen their impact and begin to get unstuck from the ruminating patterns they often put you in.

Even small shifts in understanding of thought patterns can shift a body toward greater vitality. The trick is to try to observe and challenge those thoughts as they arise. Cultivating curiosity about your mind can help your thinking feel less stuck, and this can be a useful tool in reducing anxiety. You can help your mind rewrite its internal script.

THOUGHT RECORD

Observe your thinking by using a tool called a "thought record," inspired by CBT. Start by remembering a situation in which you felt anxious. Try to reflect on other emotions you felt at that time. Then think about your thoughts. Were any of your thoughts automatic negative thoughts, or "stinking" thinking? Here is an example.

Situation	Feelings/ Emotions	Negative Automatic Thoughts	Evidence for These Thoughts	Evidence Against These Thoughts
Pain and fatigue preventing me from exercising	Anxiety Distress Resentment Fear	"I'm lazy and don't try hard enough" "I'm never getting better"	I could have exercised today if I had really pushed myself and I didn't. I have been suffering for a year and am still struggling.	I have exercised twice this week, and I need to listen to my body. I'm doing the best that I can. That's enough. I have seen progress, even if it's not as fast as I would like. It's a sign that I can continue to improve.

Turn to your journal and create your own thought record. Once you have written out your thoughts, you can examine them. Pretend you are a lawyer in the courtroom, making a case. Try to defend your thoughts. Then challenge those thoughts from the other side. How are your thoughts *not* true? Help your mind question the validity of these thoughts.

If this exercise is helping you, don't stop here. Use thought records to continue practicing. Like many other mental health tools, this exercise, if you do it regularly, can make significant changes in the way you think.

CHAPTER 13

Trauma Lives in the Body and Mind

For many people with a history of trauma, reading about trauma and traumatic experiences can be activating and destabilizing. We recommend reading this chapter in a space that feels safe and secure. Listen to your body and mind. If it feels like this chapter is activating a trauma response, allow yourself to take breaks, to practice grounding exercises, or to move to another chapter altogether. Prioritize your own well-being and engage with this chapter in any way that feels healing and supportive for you.

What You Will Learn in This Chapter:

- The signs and symptoms of trauma in long illness
- Grounding exercises and mindfulness meditations to use in trauma recovery
- Tools to help you integrate and understand parts of yourself that have been affected by trauma

I do believe that trauma can live in our bodies. In therapy, I definitely had moments where I would connect with traumatized younger parts of me. It almost felt like they came forward and said, "Hey, remember this." It was something I had forgotten. I had definitely buried it in my unconscious, never to be looked at again.

Interestingly, I had a realization that I could have a physical flare-up of my symptoms in my body, maybe from emotional stress. So I do think there is this kind of relationship between trauma and illness.

I've just decided and kind of accepted that illness is my "thing." Sometimes it is my body's way of dealing with or processing trauma.

Like a rock dropped in a pond, the ripples of traumatic experiences are felt long after the event itself.

People with a history of trauma may feel unsafe, even in a secure space. Their bodies may feel like they are on high alert. Their minds scan the environment for threats, even when they want to relax. Flashbacks and nightmares are common. Paranoia may develop for reasons they don't understand. They stay away from places or things that are related to bad memories. These things may happen only once in a while, or all the time.

If any of this is happening to you, you are probably experiencing the effects of having lived through trauma. *Trauma* is a life-threatening or harmful event or series of events that can mean different things to different people. You may have a memory of the trauma you experienced, or you might not. Details could feel fuzzy, or it may have happened too early in your life for you to remember.

In this chapter, we will not ask you to revisit past trauma directly. It is not always useful to bring up a traumatic experience without someone nearby who is directly supporting you, ideally someone with advanced training in trauma therapy. This chapter is meant to help you reflect on how past events may be impacting your emotions and your body today and to give you ideas and tools for healing from trauma moving forward.

For many people, even just reading this chapter could bring up complex and challenging emotions and physical responses in the body. Lots of people have heard the word "triggered," which is now used so much in popular culture that it isn't always meaningful. Medically, we define a "trigger" as a trauma stimulus, or a trauma reminder. Not everyone likes the word "triggered," and we invite you to use whatever term resonates most with you. A trauma stimulus can be anything from a smell to a body sensation or even a sound that brings up past trauma within you. These responses are almost always subconscious and can result in overwhelming experiences in both the mind and body. This response could look like escalating anxiety or even a panic attack, or it might lead some people to seek a space of safety, even at an inopportune moment. We know that the longer a person seeks safety and engages in avoidance, the harder it is to improve.

> *I would be sitting in class, and something would set it off. My heart would race, I would get clammy hands, I knew I needed to get out. I would leave in the middle of class and go home, curl up in bed, and watch TV. It was too much to sit with. But it wasn't good for my life.*

If this happens to you, it's not your fault. You're not trying to feel this way. We are here to give you tools for identifying a trauma stimulus and exercises to reground your mind and nervous system.

Many people feel that they are in a state of constant threat, which can bring up feelings of overwhelm, helplessness, hyperarousal, or hypoarousal. *Hyperarousal* is when the body feels too activated; you always feel on edge. People with long-standing hyperarousal feel worn out by an overactive fight-or-flight nervous system and an overworked adrenal system. *Hypoarousal* as the result of trauma can make you feel numb and disconnected from your life. It is possible to oscillate between hyper- and hypoarousal. Another possible result of trauma is *dissociation*, a feeling of being suddenly disconnected from your body and experiences, often experienced as a subconscious way to stay safe.

People with long illness may have a history of trauma before they became ill. Or they may experience trauma after becoming ill because of medical neglect, medical procedures, or hospitalizations during which they experienced life-threatening invalidation, abandonment, vulnerability, lack of control, harm, or pain with no relief. When they have symptoms of trauma while interacting with the health care system, they may be labeled as depressed or anxious when they are actually living daily with the effects of trauma. When this happens, depression and anxiety are the symptoms, not the disease. But without correct identification of what is going on with them, they are unlikely to get better.

Treatment

People living with the effects of trauma are typically treated with a combination of therapy, medication, and mindfulness. We also believe in the power of telling your story, which may include recounting trauma you have experienced, if doing so feels okay. See Chapter 23, "Your Story Is Powerful," for more information.

> **Medications and natural products:** First-line treatment is typically with the standard antidepressant medications, which can target low mood, overactivation, and anxiety. There are also medications that can address the disruptive nightmares associated with trauma (for more on nightmares, see page 146). Many of the natural products used for depression and anxiety are also used for people experiencing the effects of trauma.
>
> **Stellate ganglion block:** A stellate ganglion block is an injection into a bundle of nerves in the neck that are involved in signaling the fight-or-flight sympathetic nervous system. Typically performed by a practitioner who specializes in pain procedures, a stellate ganglion block is often covered by insurance when used to treat PTSD because of the high-quality studies supporting its use. Stellate ganglion blocks are also being used more widely in other long illnesses with autonomic dysfunction.
>
> **Therapy:** If you have been in therapy and are not getting better, you may want to consider a specialized therapy designed for healing trauma:
>
>> **Cognitive processing therapy** helps you explore and rewrite unhelpful beliefs related to past traumas.
>>
>> **Prolonged exposure therapy** helps you reprogram your response to memories, places, situations, and other cues that remind you of past trauma(s).

Eye movement desensitization and reprocessing (EMDR) helps you recall and process traumatic memories, while using eye movements to decrease the intensity of the memories.

For more help, refer to "How to Find a Therapist" (page 42). If you are unable to find a therapist, there are several workbooks on trauma that you can use to guide yourself (see the resources section).

Be Mindful of Activation of Trauma

While reading about trauma in this chapter, watch out for signs that your trauma stimulus has been activated, such as a racing heart, increased rate of breathing, chest heaviness, emotional numbness, or a sense of needing to seek immediate safety. If this comes up, consider trying the grounding exercise provided here or the safety mindfulness meditation. These can be used at any time when you start to feel your trauma response activate.

EXERCISE

GROUNDING WITH THE SENSES

Grounding can be a way to move yourself out of a trauma reaction and back into the present moment. If you are having intense emotions or a flashback, this exercise may help center and focus you in the present moment.

Sight: *Look around you. What do you see? Trying naming things. (Think of this as a game of I Spy.)*

Touch: *Feel your surroundings. Try rubbing the palms of your hands together, sliding your fingers over a surface near you, or stroking your hair.*

Sound: *Listen. What do you hear? Try to name the things you are hearing.*

Smell: *What can you smell? Take a moment to breathe deeply and see if you can pick up smells in the air.*

Taste: *What do you taste? Run your tongue around your mouth. What flavors do you notice?*

EXERCISE

MEDITATION: SAFE SPACE

You may have had the experience of becoming overwhelmed and feeling like there is nowhere you feel safe. This is a meditation for coping with that feeling.

> *Close your eyes and focus on your breath.*
>
> *Think of times when you have felt safe. This may be outdoors in nature or at the beach, or indoors on your couch. It can be either a space that you remember or a place that you create in your mind.*
>
> *Visualize yourself in this space. What does it feel like to be there? Try connecting with all of your senses in this place. Does it have sounds or smells? Can you touch the surfaces? Try to spend time in this place. Find a place to sit or lie down.*
>
> *Remember to breathe, and take five to ten minutes to be in this safe space. Remember that you can return to this space anytime that you need it.*

Journaling

SOMATIC AND EMOTIONAL INVENTORY

Think of a time in the past month when you felt a bad or traumatic memory from your past come up. What was happening in your mind at that moment? (*Note:* We are not asking you to relive the traumatic memory itself, but rather to think about your physical and emotional responses.)

How did those memories coming up affect your body? Did you notice any different sensations or feelings in your body?

Your Mind Tries to Protect You

In addition to using the tools discussed here, there are other ways to understand how trauma, traumatic experiences, and family dysfunction can affect someone with a long illness. Internal family systems (IFS) is a school of therapy that helps you understand how your internal world accommodates these experiences and allows you to have a deeper understanding and more control over how you react to and navigate in the world.

IFS outlines the ways in which the self can become fragmented when experiences are not heard or processed. Your mind has assigned different roles to different parts of yourself. No part of you is bad. They are all working for you and trying to keep you safe. But it doesn't always feel that way. Let's explore what these different parts of yourself can look like.

Core self: This is the true you. It is made up of your core attributes. Your core self can guide you through life. After a trauma, though, other parts of your system may not let it. It can be hard to experience a sense of yourself. You may feel empty, or as though you have no stable sense of identity, but like all of us, you have a core self.

Exiles: When you experience trauma and your story isn't heard or acknowledged, part of you holds on to the pain. That part of you may feel childlike and wounded. It is the most tender part of you, and it needs love, holding, and acceptance. You feel it strongly when you are triggered by things that make you feel unsafe, like invalidation around your illness or medical procedures. This part of you is the "exile" of your trauma. Your mind develops other parts of you to protect this tender part, such as managers and firefighters. A key to healing is an "unburdening" process in which the exiled part feels entirely heard, accepted, and loved by the core self and other parts.

Managers: The manager's job is to maintain control. It protects the exile part of you to ensure that you never get hurt again. The more in control the manager is, the less scary the world will be. It may decide to exert its control primarily over you. It can be a judgmental and critical inner voice. People with long illness often have overdeveloped managers and feel intense criticism from within. The manager may also manage other people by caretaking, even when you are the one who needs caretaking the most.

Firefighters: When the exile is triggered and in pain, the firefighters work to put out the fire. They jump into action, but often without thinking. They are reactive. In order to get the exile out of pain, this part of you may have you acting in ways that aren't good for you, like drinking too much, overeating, escaping situations, or engaging in self-harm. In long illness, the firefighters may be fleeing pain, rejection, and hopelessness. The firefighters do their best to get you out of discomfort, but this isn't always in line with your values for your life and health.

Journaling

Can you describe your "core self"? Is your core self able to guide you through life, or does it get overshadowed by other parts of you? How has your illness affected your ability to sense your core self?

> Do you have "exile" parts? What are they like? What are they holding on to that needs to be seen and heard?
>
> Do you have "manager" parts of yourself? How do they try to control you and your world?
>
> Do you have "firefighter" parts of yourself? If so, what do they do to try to numb your pain?

You could be feeling many different things after reading this chapter. It may have provided insight or important information to incorporate into your understanding of yourself. Maybe it has made you more aware of the tender parts of yourself (exiles) that are still feeling strongly the effects of trauma. We know that reading one chapter of a book isn't enough to address trauma. If you are resonating strongly with this chapter, we hope you will seek out more help. There are tools available to help you acknowledge trauma and heal, ideally with the support of a therapist, who can walk with you through the process. If you are unable to connect with a therapist, we recommend exploring the journals listed in the resources section.

When in doubt, move to a space where you can be safe. Try to practice one of the grounding exercises provided here, or recite the following:

"I am safer than I feel."

"It happened, it's over, I am safe now."

"This feeling is not my forever."

CHAPTER 14

Coping and State of Mind

I think the path is different for everyone on how you learn to cope. For me, I just had to think this might be my life forever. How can I make it the best life possible?

I try to talk about it like making friends with your illness, you know, treating it like a friend or at the very least, if you can't treat it like a friend, treating it like a relative—not super-exciting. You know it's the holidays, but they're still coming. I don't really like her, but I have to be cordial. If I fight with her, it's just gonna make it worse, you know, I might as well be gracious.

I think I now try to be friendly. I see it maybe now like it's a needy child. Yeah, you're having a tantrum. I see my body is having a tantrum. Okay, what would I do for a child having a tantrum right now? I would give them a quiet space, I would be nice to them. You know, I wouldn't scream at them or punish them.

What You Will Learn in This Chapter:

- How the way you cope with long illness may be helping *or* hurting you
- How your state of mind impacts the way you see the world, communicate, and make decisions
- Why it is important to balance emotional and rational thinking when making decisions in long illness

In long illness, it might seem like there is always a new issue or challenge to face. You may feel like you already have a black belt in coping, but you can always learn a few more moves!

Most of us use both helpful and harmful coping strategies. People do best when they have a mix of positive coping strategies. As you read through the following list of common helpful and harmful coping skills, think about the coping strategies you use.

Helpful Coping Strategies

- **Emotional release.** Feel your feelings—scream, yell, or cry.
- **Do something creative.** Try drawing, writing, or dancing.
- **Use mindfulness.** Try a five-minute guided meditation app or progressive muscle relaxation (see the resources section for more ideas on mindfulness).
- **Find a distraction.** Watch a TV show, read a book, or call a friend.
- **Try self-soothing.** Use your five senses to manage your stress. Give yourself a hug (gently cross your arms at your chest and hold), take a bubble bath, drink a warm beverage, or try self-massage. (See page 108 for self-massage.)
- **Challenge your thoughts.** Balance your negative thoughts with opposite thoughts. See Chapter 12 on anxiety and stinking thinking for more information; try completing a thought record exercise.
- **Ask for help.** Call a friend or family member, or reach out to your health care practitioner.
- **Get yourself grounded.** Try being in nature. Take your shoes off in the grass and notice all of your senses.
- **Write in your journal.** Record your thoughts, feelings, and experiences.
- **Set boundaries.** There are times when we need to say "no." Remember that "No" can be a full sentence.
- **Adjust your body temperature.** If you are stressed, you may be feeling hot. Try splashing cold water on your face or holding an ice pack on your neck.
- **Exercise.** Move your body.

Harmful Coping Strategies

- Getting stuck in your head: Worrying, catastrophizing
- Feeling overly responsible and guilty
- Avoidance: Staying away from situations that bring up hard feelings or feel scary
- Oversleeping
- Undersleeping
- Eating to self-soothe, overeating in large quantities, or repeatedly reaching for foods that don't agree with you, bringing up feelings of guilt and shame
- Undereating
- Unloading negative emotions onto others or taking your stress out on another person
- Heavy alcohol intake (initially relaxing, but a slippery slope to use as a primary coping strategy)
- Using recreational drugs
- Self-harm

Note: As with so many things, advice can seem like nothing more than platitudes. We know it's often not easy to ask for help, let alone recognize when you might have a problem, especially with alcohol, drugs, food restriction, or self-harm. You've been through so much with long illness, but sometimes the coping mechanisms that make you feel better in the short run can do long-term damage. We encourage you to be kind and gentle with yourself. If you think one of your coping strategies has become problematic, try journaling to concretize your feelings, and then seek out professional help. Seeking help is not a sign of weakness. You are worth love, care, and support.

Journaling

MY COPING MECHANISMS

Look at the list of coping strategies and write down all of the ones that apply to you.

Now write the top four coping mechanisms you would like to try to use.

Example:

Coping mechanism: Ask for help

What would this look like? I call my aunt who is a good listener, or leave a message for my therapist.

Journaling

COPING WITH STRESS

Think about a stressful time in your life and try to remember the coping strategies that you used. Were they helpful, harmful, or both? If you have a similar issue in the future, what is one new strategy you could try? How might using that strategy change the experience?

States of Mind

The mind shifts in and out of different states from one day to the next, dictating your thoughts and behaviors. Shifting your state of mind can make your thinking clearer. We have found that states of mind are particularly important to consider in long illness because of their impact on the vital decisions you are faced with every day about your health and eventual recovery.

In long illness, anxiety, shame, pain, and resentment can all cloud your thinking. Some people can become so overwhelmed by their current situation that they shut down their emotions altogether. Neither ignoring your emotions or giving them free rein is helpful for moving toward your goals and values around your health. This is particularly true when you're accessing health care: being able to think clearly about your medical appointments, medical decisions, and communication with your health care team is essential to recovery.

For example, in anticipation of a medical appointment, you may have questions about your symptoms and experiences. But when you get to the office, you clam up. You feel chest tightness and hear an inner voice saying, *The doctor doesn't want to hear it, don't complain.* This is an emotional thought process driven by fear—and maybe by past experiences. If you stay quiet and don't tell the practitioner what you've been experiencing, that would be a decision made purely out of emotion, without bringing in the rational part of your brain that knows you need to tell your practitioner what is going on before they can try to help you.

Making decisions purely out of your emotions can be self-defeating. The same is true for making purely rational decisions that don't take into account your emotional truth.

Dialectical behavioral therapy (DBT) focuses on the three states of mind that most of us go in and out of. The long-term goal is to be able to spend more time in "wise mind," which gives us more access to our intellect and feelings at the same time.

	Description	*Behaviors*	*Thoughts*
Emotional mind: "I want"	Your emotions are running the show. Facts and intellect don't play a part in your actions and responses.	You often act impulsively, without considering consequences. *Example:* Road rage	Your emotionally charged thinking is black-and-white, with no shades of gray. *Examples:* "They hate me"; "I'm bad"; "They're awful."
Rational mind: "I should"	You are using your intellect only. Your feelings are not part of the equation. Facts alone rule your thoughts and decisions, with no consideration for what you want or how you feel.	You often act out of obligation, while not always pursuing something you actually want. *Example:* You take on a new responsibility because it's the "right thing to do," without acknowledging how overwhelmed you might feel.	In rational mind thinking, you are "should-ing" all over yourself. *Example:* "I should pick him up from the airport, even if I'm busy"; "I shouldn't go out to dinner because it's cheaper to eat at home."

Wise mind: "I balance"	You weigh both facts and emotions. You consider the bigger picture and examine a problem from many angles to balance the emotional and rational factors.	You make decisions that are less impulsive and more in line with your values. *Example:* You know you *should* exercise, but you are tired. You do a five-minute yoga practice, then rest.	You observe the relationship between your thoughts and emotions and try to weigh both. *Example:* In a state of wise mind, the thought "She didn't say hello to me because she hates me" shifts to "She didn't say hello. She may not like me, but it's more likely that she is busy and distracted."

Journaling

Reflect on two recent decisions you made. Were they made with your emotional mind, rational mind, or wise mind? What was the result of this decision? Would you like to do anything differently in the future?

In long illness, many things are beyond your control. Coping strategies and states of mind are concepts that *can* shift your experience, regardless of the current state of your health. With reflection and self-awareness, cultivating these skills can make a big difference. When you cope in healthier ways, you aren't depleting your energy reserves but actually are replenishing them. Reflecting on your state of mind before you make a decision about your health could make your choices clearer. Making sure that you are in a wise mind before engaging in a conversation with your partner or friend could preserve a relationship.

This form of healing is an inside job, and it's worth the extra time it takes to understand and shift strategies or states of mind where you can. Your body and mind will thank you.

PART IV

LONG-TERM SOLUTIONS AND LIFESTYLE MEDICINE

In my experience, when I make one positive lifestyle change, it creates a cascade of other positive changes. I see in myself, when I exercise, I'm more likely to eat well, and I'm more likely to sleep well at night and fall asleep. It's all related. When I am able to make a choice that is good for my body, other decisions and choices more easily fall into place. I make more positive choices, and I am much better able to deal with problems as they come up.

Lifestyle medicine aims to prevent, treat, and reverse chronic illness by encouraging pro-health, anti-inflammatory behaviors. While some of this information may seem obvious, the evidence behind it is strong. The chapters on stress, nutrition, movement, and sleep will introduce you to the evidence behind many of the things your grandmother already told you were good for you.

We realize that the thought of changing your lifestyle may seem stressful and overwhelming because, well, "lifestyle" is everything you do every day in order to survive, and it is exhausting to think about how you might need to change it all. One big reminder here: these chapters are not meant to make you feel frustrated or guilty. For some of you, changing your routine is simply not an option right now. We see you. Hang in there. This information is here for you to visit when you are ready. For those of you who are willing and able to make many changes right away, try to start slowly to set yourself up for success. We do not recommend making multiple big changes all at once because, even if they are changes in the right direction, change brings stress. The choices you make every second contribute to your health. Revisiting this book often will allow you to make more small changes to layer on top of your other anti-inflammatory behaviors.

CHAPTER 15

Your Body's Detox System

I got to this point where I would have tried anything that would have made my body feel better. I wanted to get the "bad stuff" out. I tried juice cleanses, teas, supplements, and different diet plans aimed at removing all the "bad stuff" that had built up in my body from being sick. Eventually I realized it wasn't about doing extreme things to get the "bad stuff" out, but to make better choices about how much "bad stuff" I was bringing into my body. I had to start being more thoughtful about how I treated myself, from what I put in my mouth to the people I surrounded myself with. Everything counts.

What You Will Learn in This Chapter:

- An overview of your body's innate power to detoxify
- Strategies for reducing your body's toxic burden
- Integrative tools for helping you clear toxins and support vitality

Your body is constantly exposed to *toxins*—the harmful substances that are in food, water, medications, supplements, air, and the environment. Toxins are in our floor cleaners and our face products, our couches and our paints. Your body itself makes toxic by-products during metabolism, such as free radicals. With long illness, your body is already working overtime to break down medications and tamp down inflammation. Every stressor, including toxins you expose yourself to, adds more work for your body. In long illness, reducing those stressors can leave you with just a little bit more energy to get through the day.

It is tempting to think you can somehow clean out your organs, ridding them of all the bad stuff they have been exposed to—and there is a whole industry that caters to long illness sufferers, promising that detoxification will lead to health—but that is not how it works. Your body does an excellent job of detoxing itself.

We would like you to meet your detox team: the liver, kidneys, colon, lymphatic system, skin, and lungs. These systems work together in a process to get toxins out, keep them out, and keep your body working well.

Step 1: Neutralize!

Your primary detoxification site is your liver, which neutralizes toxins using a system of more than fifty enzymes that break down chemicals. This function is important to people with a long illness because they might be exposed to more chemicals and medications than their non-ill peers and therefore have a higher toxic burden. There might be genetic differences in this system for some people with drug sensitivities (for example, drugs have a stronger, longer effect on them, or drugs wear off quickly).

This is why your pharmacist sometimes warns you not to take certain medications with others, and why some medication doses have to be adjusted. To avoid adverse interactions, it is essential for you to tell all your practitioners about all of the medications, supplements, adaptogens, and chemicals that you are putting into your body. A natural supplement that you think is safe can make a medication ineffective or even toxic. (See Chapter 21 on natural supplements.)

"Great," you might be thinking, "so my liver can neutralize all the bad stuff that I take in." Unfortunately, the liver can only do so much! The proteins that break down toxins are available in a limited supply, and some of the substances you take in can also cause liver damage. Your liver has a key antioxidant that helps protect it from toxic damage: glutathione. Many people with high levels of stress from chronic disease don't have enough glutathione to protect their liver from damage. Sometimes liver damage is so bad that the cells die.

TIPS

How to Increase Your Glutathione
- **Eat foods rich in glutathione:** Avocados, spinach, and asparagus.
- **Eat foods that support glutathione supplies:** Brussels sprouts, cauliflower, broccoli, kale, and mustard greens; garlic, shallots, and onions; fish and poultry.
- **Eat foods high in cysteine** (a building block needed to make glutathione): eggs, sunflower seeds, beans, and whey; citrus fruits, kiwi, and peppers; Brazil nuts, fish, cottage cheese, and brown rice. Cysteine can also be taken as a natural product called N-acetylcysteine (NAC).
- **Eat foods high in vitamin C** (which helps turn on glutathione and can help reduce toxic damage): citrus fruits, kiwi, and peppers.
- **Eat foods with selenium** (a key component of glutathione): Brazil nuts, fish, cottage cheese, and brown rice. (*Note:* Get selenium from food sources, since high levels of selenium from supplements can have the opposite effect!)
- **Cut out or reduce alcohol:** Alcohol uses a large percentage of your glutathione.
- **Get regular, high-quality sleep and exercise:** Both good sleep and exercise increase your glutathione levels.

Be cautious when using natural products and other ways of increasing glutathione. Glutathione has been shown to increase when people supplement their diets with milk thistle and turmeric, but as with all supplements, consult your practitioners before taking them. Oral glutathione is not well absorbed and is not a great way to increase your levels. We do not recommend trying to increase your glutathione level with intravenous (IV) glutathione, often available at IV infusion centers. There isn't enough evidence to support its use medically. And IV glutathione doesn't meet our threshold for safety, as placing an IV puts you at risk of infection and damage to your blood vessels. As with all new medications or natural products, you should talk with your care team to see if trying supplements to increase your glutathione levels would be useful for you and if it is safe for you.

Step 2: Eliminate

Your liver has neutralized the toxin and changed it to a form that can be expelled through your urine by the kidneys or through your feces. Here are the body systems that are key to this phase:

Kidneys: Your kidneys filter all the blood in your body and need adequate hydration to filter and eliminate the toxins. Drinking at least two to three liters of water per day can support toxin elimination.

Colon: Your colon absorbs water and expels solid waste as feces. Many people are constipated owing to lack of adequate hydration, low fiber, and an unbalanced gut microbiome.

Lymphatic system: Lymph nodes and the channels that connect them are known as your lymphatic system. They travel alongside your blood supply, are in all parts of your body, and help clear infections. During infections, they can become enlarged and sometimes hurt. Aside from good hydration, your lymphatic system thrives when the body sweats. When the lymphatic system is blocked or is having difficulty flowing, lymph swelling (lymphedema) can develop. Lymphatic massage is often prescribed to people who have experienced surgeries or injuries around lymph nodes, which could be impairing lymphatic drainage. There is good evidence that lymphatic drainage can improve multiple symptoms and quality of life for people experiencing cancer, fibromyalgia, and IBS constipation. (See page 209 for a lymphatic release exercise.)

Skin: Your skin releases toxins by sweating. Exercise that makes you sweat is great, because perspiration has benefits throughout your body. Other means of sweating also are beneficial. Warm Epsom salt (or Dead Sea salt/magnesium) baths, saunas (dry or infrared), or sitting in the hot sun wrapped in a towel (to avoid the UV radiation) are great ways to get your skin detox system ramped up, if you can tolerate increased heat.

Lungs: Your lungs are constantly filtering out toxins from the outside, such as dust in your home, pollution, or chemicals. They do a great job on their own. If you smoke in any form—tobacco, natural herbs, marijuana, hookah, vaping—it's important to stop, because there are many toxins that overload your lungs when you smoke. Your lungs are more prone to long-term damage from smoking when you are chronically ill. The only thing that should be inhaled into your lungs besides air is medication prescribed by a practitioner.

To keep your lungs in good condition, check the air quality in your location daily and change your activities based on the recommendations (when air quality is poor, you might want to stay inside and not exercise heavily). Many people with lung disease, allergies, or chronic illness should consider investing in quality air filters. Often pollution indoors is worse than the outdoor air owing to the buildup of dust and dirt, carbon monoxide, ozone, and volatile organic compounds, which can worsen underlying lung conditions.

Your Toxic Load

If your body already has an amazing built-in detox system that is doing a great job, why do you feel so bad? Reducing toxin exposure is the key to supporting your detox system. Let's check your toxin load to see how you are doing.

Journaling

TOXIN INVENTORY

Following is a list of common toxins, substances, and activities that might be overloading your detox system. In one column, write down and check those that you are able to decrease your exposure to; in another column, write down and circle those that you can't change.

Alcohol	Smoking	Recreational drugs
Medications	Supplements and vitamins	Tainted drinking water
Caffeine	High-salt diet	Dehydration
Processed foods	Refined vegetable and seed oils	Trans fats
Loud sounds	Bright light at night	Bug repellants
High-fructose corn syrup	Grilled and smoked meat	Added sugar
Mercury (in some seafood)	Dioxins (in fatty meat, dairy)	Pesticides and herbicides
Lead (in water)	Arsenic (in water, rice, chicken)	Nonstick coatings
Air pollution	Asbestos	Fabric softeners
Beauty products	Plastics (e.g., bisphenol A [BPA])	Glycol ethers (dry cleaning)
Flame retardants	Chemical solvents	Cleaning products

What toxin sources in this list stand out to you?

What areas in your life can you improve on?

TIPS

Decrease Your Toxin Load

Decreasing your toxin load is the most important way to detox. It is more important and effective than any detox product you can buy or detox protocol you could follow, hands down.

- **Hydrate.** Your detox systems cannot work well when you are low on water. You need to drink more water. Not sparkling water, not soda, not coffee—just plain water! You can add some lemon if that helps get you in the habit. Start with 2.7 liters (91 ounces) daily for women and 3.7 liters (125 ounces) daily for men. This is the minimum. If you are exercising, you need more water, especially before (half a liter two hours before) and during exercise (to replace loss, depending on how much you sweat). Check out your local water company's website for information about the quality of your water. For most of us, tap water is safe. Some people use a water filtration system, which can remove more potential toxins from water. Do your research before investing in such a system to make sure you are getting a product worth paying for. For more about hydration, see Chapter 17.

- **Check your produce.** Choose organic produce if possible and wash all of your produce (even organic!) to remove debris and toxins. Not all produce is exposed to pesticides at the same rate. Make sure you water-wash the "Dirty Dozen" culprits in your produce aisle: strawberries, spinach, kale, collard and mustard greens, nectarines, apples, grapes, cherries, peaches, pears, bell and hot peppers, celery, and tomatoes. Check out "Good Food on a Tight Budget" from the Environmental Working Group (www.ewg.org/goodfood), which provides ways to save money while optimizing your diet.

- **Target a healthy weight.** You aren't sick only because of your weight, and your weight is not a reflection of your worth. But we know that for people who are overweight, reducing fat stores can reduce strain on the liver and support optimal detoxification.

- **Stop or reduce smoking, alcohol consumption, use of medications or supplements you do not need or are not prescribed, and use of recreational drugs.** Ideally, you want to reduce your body's exposure to anything that moves it away from vitality, especially substances that are hard on the detoxification systems in your body. The pain and distress of long illness can send you looking for relief through drinking, smoking, recreational drugs, or misuse of prescribed medications. With long illness, however, these kinds of substances can take an even greater toll on your body. Because of the level of discomfort and distress in long illness, it is easy to develop an unhealthy relationship with substances; you may be using them more often than you would like, or having health consequences from using them but being unable to stop. Talk to your primary practitioner about your relationship to substances if you are concerned, especially if you are noting health consequences. A host of resources, including medications and psychotherapy, are available to help you reduce your use. For more information, visit the Substance Abuse and Mental Health Services Administration website (www.samhsa.gov) or call the US National Helpline (1-800-662-4357 or TTY 1-800-487-4889 24/7/365). If you are thinking about quitting smoking or want support, call 1-800-QUIT-NOW (784-8669) to speak with counselors who can support you.

- **Avoid and reduce your use of items known to have a high toxin load.** Although your body is amazing at clearing out most toxins you ingest or are exposed to, it doesn't get everything. You might have noticed that more of the products you buy are labeled "organic," "non-toxic," or "BPA-free." Researchers have found that certain chemicals have serious effects on our health, and many of them are being removed from foods and other products, sometimes voluntarily and sometimes to follow government rules. We're not suggesting that you cut out all of your favorite things, just that you think more about little steps you can take to reduce your toxin burden. Those little steps will add up.

TIPS

Reduce Toxin Exposure at Home

- Take off your shoes at the door to avoid tracking in debris from the outside.
- Dust, vacuum, and mop regularly to keep down levels of dust.
- Swap out chemical-laden cleaners for natural ones. Vinegar and baking soda can go a long way in keeping your home clean and are very cheap.
- Use less plastic, especially for your food. When you can, swap out plastic for glass, ceramic, or stainless steel. Reuse glass jars from other foods for storage and do not heat food in plastic containers or on plastic plates. When it's time to replace your cookware, swap out nonstick pans, which are coated in plastics, for cast iron or stainless steel. Buy products labeled "BPA-free," including canned foods and beverages.
- Choose safer home improvement products, such as low-EVO paint at the hardware store.
- Consider toxin-free or toxin-reduced products when buying furniture, bedding, and other items for your home.
- Avoid dry cleaning when possible. Use green dry cleaners if necessary, and consider steam as an option.

- Cut down on scented air fresheners, candles, and perfumes, as they often have high levels of toxins. Look into natural or essential oils if you desire fragrance, but remember that these can irritate some people and should be used with caution in a home with children.
- Look for consumer guides for cleaning products, foods, personal products, water, and more to learn further about toxin-reducing changes.

To reduce your body and home toxin loads, check out the Environmental Working Group (www.ewg.org) for great tips and suggestions. It's not realistic to eliminate everything that is bad, but just swapping some of your products for less toxic ones will make a significant difference.

Detox FAQs

Do I need to do a liver detox? While PMS, hormone imbalances, bloating, gas, poor sleep, and allergies can be signs that your oxidative stress levels are high and your liver needs a break, we do not have the data to recommend a commercial liver cleanse, which hasn't been proven to work.

These symptoms also occur with many conditions that have nothing to do with the liver. It is good to look at your detoxification system and think about how you might be overloading it, but a typical detox product is not the answer. Need more reminders why?

- Your body already is doing a good job detoxing you.
- The best thing to do is to reduce your toxic load.
- Many detox teas and supplements are unregulated, have side effects and toxins themselves, and cost money, and there is limited evidence that they are effective.
- Extreme dieting and caloric restriction can cause oxidative stress, decreasing the body's ability to naturally detox.

Do I need a colonic to flush my colon? We do not recommend these for patients with chronic conditions because there are many side effects. Cramping, bloating, diarrhea, nausea, dehydration, tears in the rectum, electrolyte imbalances, and infections can be disastrous for those already juggling other symptoms. Instead of a colonic, try to drink more water, move around, eat an anti-inflammatory diet high in fiber, and ensure that you're having regular bowel movements.

If you are still interested in a colonic, please check with your health care team first, as they may have specific recommendations or concerns about your unique body. Make sure to get a list of ingredients in the colonic for your practitioner so they can advise you if it is medically safe for your condition.

Should I use a sauna to detox? Saunas are a great way to sweat and release toxins that might have been absorbed into the top layer of your skin. While your liver and kidneys do most of the work of getting toxins out, a small amount of metal comes out in sweat. Both infrared and dry saunas also have health benefits beyond detoxification. Heat therapy drops your blood pressure, decreases inflammation, decreases free radical and oxidative stress, and improves the function of your immune system. Using a dry sauna more than four times weekly is associated with a significant decrease in stroke, dementia, and Alzheimer's disease. Studies of infrared, low-temperature saunas also look promising. Other studies have suggested that sauna use improves shortness of breath, recovery after exercise, fibromyalgia pain, chronic fatigue syndrome, and depression.

Most of us don't have easy access to a sauna. You can now buy a home sauna unit or sauna blanket, and you can also find saunas in gyms, bathhouses, and cultural centers that are free or low-cost.

Check with your practitioner to discuss whether heat therapy is safe for your condition.

Journaling

THE PHYSICAL TOXINS IN YOUR LIFE

Revisit the toxin inventory on page 203. Are there certain areas of your life where you could try to reduce your toxic load? What are one or two ways you could reduce your toxic load this week? When will you try it? How long will you try a new behavior for?

EXERCISE

LYMPHATIC RELEASE AND DRAINAGE

Dry brushing is a healing practice ritual in Ayurvedic medicine that is used to stimulate circulation and promote lymphatic flow and drainage. To dry brush, you need a firm-bristled brush or a dry hand towel. Avoid broken or damaged skin, and don't brush your face. There is minimal harm in trying dry brushing, but skip it if you have a skin condition or sensitive skin.

Note: Lymphatic release is usually very safe, comfortable, and pleasurable. But you should discuss it with your practitioners first if you have a medical condition such as heart, liver, or kidney disease or a history of blood clots or strokes. Do not try dry brushing if you have an infection. Your practitioners can tell you how to optimize these relaxation and drainage techniques based on your limitations.

Dry Brushing

Start at your feet with your brush or towel. Stroke your skin with long, fluid, light swipes, going up toward your heart until you get to your belly. You might see faint red marks that should not hurt, and they should not linger for long. Stroke gently on your abdomen and back toward your heart; this skin might be more sensitive than your legs. Next go to your hands and stroke toward your heart.

Lymphatic Stimulation

You can also try lymphatic self-massage. There are many different areas you can concentrate on, depending on your body and your goals. We suggest that you release the skin at the front of your neck, which promotes the lymph fluid that drains to your heart (back into your main circulation). Place your index and middle fingers flat on the top of your collarbone by your shoulder. Keeping your fingers above your collarbone, gently glide your flat fingers down toward the middle of your neck, tracing the top of your collarbone and maintaining a slight tug on the skin. You should feel the skin on your neck gently stretching, but this should not be painful, and you should not dig with your fingertips. Stretch the skin as far as you can without pain—perhaps to the end of the collarbone—then let it go. Repeat on each side fifteen times.

Finishing Up

Whichever form of lymphatic release you perform, you can finish the same way:

> *Shower with warm water. Towel off.*
>
> *Apply moisturizing oil to your body (coconut oil, for example) with your hands, starting at your limbs and rubbing toward your heart (similar to how you brushed).*
>
> *Lie down and rest for ten minutes. Take deep breaths during this time and enjoy some gentle stretches on your back.*

Mental Detox

Our minds are stimulated every day by everything in our environment, our interactions, and our thoughts, both good and bad. Excess mental toxins can make you feel stagnant, overloaded, anxious, and even demoralized. There is no way to avoid all bad things in your life, and stress in small doses isn't bad for you. But if you are repeatedly finding yourself in stressful, negative situations, your mind can get overloaded. A mental detox will push pause on day-to-day distractions, anxieties, and stressors.

Journaling

PRIORITIZE YOUR ENERGY

Since your energy is limited, who or what should get it? With long illness, you already have a bit more to manage than you used to. Use your journal to take an inventory of the things in your life that strengthen your mental energy and those things that decrease it.

Begin by reflecting on people and activities in your life that build you up, charge your energy, make you feel alive and vital, and usually bring you joy. These are activities you are happy to do and people who make you feel supported. What activities in your life are like this? Are there areas in your life that make you feel light, happy, joyous, strong, valued, and seen? What activities do you want to spend more time doing? Who supports your detoxification and clarity?

Now reflect on people and activities that bring you down or drain your energy. Someone you think of might not drain you all the time but only in certain situations, like in work meetings, or while making decisions about household chores. Scan the list here. Do any of these areas of life feel toxic, heavy, draining, overwhelming, or too stressful to you? What do you dread, avoid, or hate for no good reason? What overloads your circuits? What could you let go of or reduce to boost your vitality? What would allow you to emotionally detoxify?

Let's take an inventory of things in your life that strengthen or decrease your mental energy. "Environments" can include social, political, and physical issues, smells, safety concerns, and many other aspects of your life. "Relationships" refers to the people you interact with in those environments.

Create two columns in your journal: one for what is healthy and strengthening, and one for what is unhealthy and depleting. Now consider these topics and relationships, writing down what is strengthening and what is depleting about each:

Living environment	Work environment	News
Friends	Work relationships	Self-expectations
Family	Community	Self-image
Intimate partners	Technology	Self-esteem
Caregivers	Social media	Thought patterns

Journaling

REFLECTING ON MENTAL DETOX

Reflect first on the list you just created of the healthy things in your life that strengthen your ability to emotionally detoxify.

> What about these relationships builds you up? Do you notice a pattern?
>
> What can you do in the coming days to increase the amount of time you are exposed to something that makes you feel more resilient in the face of mental stressors?

> Write one goal for the week.
>
> After a week passes, reflect on how making the change to attain that goal made you feel. If your feeling was positive, how can you sustain this change in your life?
>
> Next reflect on the list of what depletes you. This list can be overwhelming. You can't be expected to change these all at once, but it is helpful to be aware of some of the things that stress you out so much that they negatively affect your health—for example, a work deadline, an unresolved conflict with someone, an ailing loved one, financial pressures, or procrastinating on tasks that need to be done. Awareness is the first step.
>
> Aside from increasing activity in areas that build you up, we also want you to pick one thing that feels mentally toxic to you, or that exhausts you. If possible, pick one that might be easy to change. Always start with the easiest.
>
> How could you reduce that stressor this week? Try to make that change and then return here to reflect on whether it helped or not. If it did, can you make it sustainable? If it did not, is there another approach you could take? Or another stressor you could work on instead?

EXERCISE

MINDFULNESS: "KEEP IN, LEAVE OUT"

This simple breathing exercise will allow your mind to reflect on what is contributing to your vitality and worth keeping, and what can be released.

Sit in a quiet place with your palms resting on your knees or beside you if you are lying down. Start by taking long deep breaths. On the inhale, close your hands into fists and ask yourself, "What do I keep in?" Imagine all the strengthening things in your life flowing in with your breath. On the exhale, open your hands and stretch your fingers. Ask yourself, "What do I leave out?" As you exhale, imagine the mental stressors you do not need flowing out in your breath and moving farther and farther away from you.

There don't need to be answers to these questions. Let your mind wander as you breathe and recite these phrases in your mind or out loud.

CHAPTER 16

Reduce Your Stress

I have a busy life. Sometimes work or the kids can be very demanding of my time. I would say, "I am so stressed." At times I was exhausted, but I could keep my head above water. Sometimes the stress even felt exhilarating and pushed me to do more.

When I started to get sick, I felt any sense of control slipping away from me. It took every ounce of energy just to take care of myself, and sometimes I needed others to help me with that. While I eventually got much better, I still have times I am sick, and the amount of stress in my life goes from doable to complete shutdown instantly. Now I see things in my life as possible stressors instead of opportunities for adventure. I have learned tricks to build up my stress tolerance, but I also have learned what helps me reduce my stress levels. For me, building a community with other moms with health challenges was great. We meet three times a week at the park, and if someone can't make it, we take turns watching each other's kids. It has built community and also gives me a break and my kids a chance to keep playing while I get some rest.

Similar to inflammation, stress is a natural defense response. Stress can help you build resilience and strength, but long-term stress or high levels of stress turn on systemic inflammation, which leads to chronic disease. With long illness, you probably already have more physical and mental stressors in your life than average, so any extra stress can tip you over the edge.

Some sources of stress are out of your direct control, but others can be reframed and approached using mindfulness and other techniques. You can regain power when you learn your triggers and address stress before or while it is happening.

What You Will Learn in This Chapter:

- The difference between good stress and bad stress
- Why chronic stress is so bad
- The effects of stress on your body and its effects on long illness
- Practices to reduce stress

Stress—Is It Really Good for You?

Imagine that you have to give a talk to a community group about something important. This prospect makes most people's muscles tighten or stomach churn. It's supposed to. Small amounts of pressure give you just the right amount of stress you need to perform at your best.

Each of us has unique responses to stress. From your awareness of threat to how your brain perceives it and how your brain and body react, there are hundreds of steps that result in a single reaction to a stressor. Each reaction is an opportunity for your brain to learn about stress. How you deal with each stressor, consciously and unconsciously, teaches your body how to respond to the next stressor. And depending on how much stress you experience and how big a threat it is to your sense of safety, your body may respond more in certain situations.

If you have a long illness, extra stress can overload you faster and push you into a state of illness. We want to help you identify your unique stress profile and how you can avoid setting off flares of your illness.

How Is Chronic Stress Different?

We often are juggling multiple stressors, and sometimes our bodies eventually become overloaded. The stress response generates free radicals, the damaging particles that lead to inflammation (see Chapter 18). There is a limit to what we can withstand individually, and to what the human body can withstand.

The total burden on your body that builds up as you are exposed to repeated stressors is referred to as *allostatic load*. Stress chemicals released from your sympathetic nervous system and adrenal hormone system protect your body from the effects of stress at low levels. The problem comes at high levels. If exposed to stress repeatedly over time, your body can be overloaded, resulting in the physiological consequences, like disease, of inflammation caused by free radicals. Over time chronic stress can lead to an inability to feel pleasure, avoidance of social situations, metabolism changes, and many other disease states.

The graph here illustrates what happens: Exposed to low amounts of stress, you might be unmotivated to do tasks, but as pressure is applied you perform your best. As the load of stress continues to increase, however, your performance markedly declines, and eventually you're unable to complete tasks.

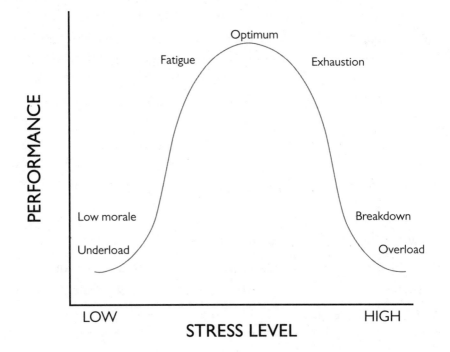

Chronic stress and related emotional states can lead to dysfunctional mitochondria. Long-term changes begin in reaction to chronic stress, including increased inflammation, changes in the size and function of areas of the brain, and changes in gene and epigenome expression. These changes cause your cells to age at a faster rate.

The aging of cells is measured by the length of your telomeres. Imagine your DNA as a shoelace: the telomeres are the caps at the end that protect the DNA from breaking down. As we age we lose some of our protective telomeres, and the DNA can get damaged. This is part of normal aging. However, people with higher levels of stress have shorter telomeres, and sometimes one stressful year can equal five to ten average stressful years.

Although some people wear their resilience to stress as a badge of pride, there is a reason it is called "the silent killer." The effects of stress can be especially damaging if you have long illness. You may think you can handle the stress you put on yourself, but it is doing long-term damage to your body when you don't take breaks, rest in between stressful events, and continue to work on developing and building your coping skills and resilience.

What's Happening Inside Your Body When You're Stressed

When your body detects emotional or physical stress, your sympathetic nervous system is activated. Your brain releases chemical signals that cause an increase in adrenaline (epinephrine) and cortisol in your blood. These two big stress hormones are made and released by the adrenal gland, which sits by your kidneys. Adrenaline increases your heart rate, your breathing rate, and your carbohydrate metabolism so that you can use energy quickly in case you need to run away. Cortisol gets sugar into the bloodstream by increasing its production so that your brain can have ample energy to get you out of harm's way. Cortisol also sends a message to your digestive, reproductive, and immune systems to stop using as much energy.

These systems are great in an emergency, but when you are under chronic stress, the effect on them can be serious. For people with long illness, the following symptoms can feel all too familiar:

WHAT HAPPENS IN THE ORGAN SYSTEMS UNDER STRESS

Respiratory	Your rate of breathing increases to get more oxygen into your blood. If the rate increases too much, the result can be hyperventilation, which is sometimes seen in anxiety or panic attacks.
Cardiovascular	Your heart rate and blood pressure increase in the short term. Over time, damage can increase your risk of hypertension, heart attack, and stroke.
Gastrointestinal	Stress interferes with the normal release of digestive enzymes, food digestion, absorption of nutrients, and elimination of waste. Symptoms can include heartburn, reflux, poor absorption, stomach pain, bloating, nausea, diarrhea, and constipation.
Immune	Fewer immune cells are made, increasing the risk of infections and worsening chronic inflammation. Immune cells in the brain trigger inflammation, which can cause depression and anxiety-like symptoms.
Endocrine	Stress hormone release can increase the risk of diabetes, decrease sperm production, decrease testosterone in men, change the menstrual cycle, and worsen PMS symptoms.
Musculoskeletal	Your muscles tense, causing aches, headaches, and body pain.
Nervous	Difficulty sleeping, inability to pay attention, learning difficulties, memory problems, mood swings, or irritability. Over the long term, the amygdala (the part of your brain that governs fear) enlarges, and the hippocampus and prefrontal cortex (memory and decision-making) shrink.

Reducing Stress

Stress reduction practices can decrease inflammation and noticeably reduce symptoms, especially over time with routine practice. Even moments of micro-relaxation can turn down your stress levels. Mindfulness, stress management classes, education about stress, breathing exercises, yoga, exercise, dietary changes, and practicing self-compassion are all ways to take good care of your mitochondrial health. Having plans for when things get difficult is key in reducing the effects of stress. Ask your practitioners if stress-reduction classes or apps are available through your care system.

EXERCISE

TIPS TO REDUCE YOUR STRESS

Here is a list of common techniques that reduce stress. In your journal, create three columns. In the first, write down the techniques you use. In the second, write down the ones you want to try. In a third column, write down what else you do to relieve stress or calm yourself in stressful situations.

Be in nature	Journal	Talk to a friend	Hug someone
Deep breathing	Take a break	Do aromatherapy	Call in sick
Listen to music	Meditate	Exercise	Laugh
Read	Do a crossword	Knit	Watch TV
Walk	Take a bath	Make a to-do list	Stretch

Mindfulness

We introduced mindfulness, the practice of being aware in the present moment, in Chapter 1, but it's worth focusing on mindfulness explicitly here for stress reduction. Right now, focus on the environment around you, the chair you are sitting in, the book in your hand, the smell of the air, the sounds you hear. Observe your thoughts. Pause. This is mindfulness. Each step, each breath, focuses on that second. When thoughts like planning for the future or dwelling on the past pop into your head—which is common and should happen—bring your focus back to the present moment.

If you have a long illness, mindfulness helps you become more aware of your body. By being more tuned in, you become more sensitive to when you start to feel symptoms of stress and can respond by turning down your stress sooner. Mindfulness practice can help you decrease your sensations

of pain, heart rate, blood pressure, cognitive decline from aging, inflammatory markers, and other effects of aging. It can reduce symptoms of anxiety
and depression and improve your self-esteem and quality of life.

Many medical centers offer a mindfulness-based stress reduction (MBSR)
course, or you can take a course online. Some of these courses have a cost,
but some are offered free for certain conditions or at certain centers. There
are many smartphone apps, books, and other media that are free or low-
cost and can help you get started with mindfulness. (See the resources on
pages 331–338.)

Seek Out Social Support

For most people, long illness goes hand in hand with some degree of loneliness. Many people with "differences," including people with long illness,
those with a disability, immigrants, the LGBTQIA+ population, and the
elderly, experience higher levels of loneliness than average. Over one-third
of adults feel lonely and one-fourth of adults over age sixty-five have no
social connections. Loneliness is bad for your health, increasing your mortality risk by 25 percent and putting you at a higher risk of cognitive decline,
dementia, and depression.

Moving toward connecting with other people can be healing but may
not always be possible if you are exhausted or in pain. Tell someone on your
medical team or in your community about the loneliness you experience
as the result of your illness. You can also explore some of these options for
increasing social connections:

Join a support group or interest group
Take a class
Get a pet or take care of a friend's pet
Volunteer with an organization you are interested in
Sign up to do something in your community, such as a volunteer cleanup
   day or reading books to children
Ask your mental health practitioner about therapy groups

Talk to strangers, say hi to neighbors, strike up a conversation with a
person you pass on the street

Schedule quality time to spend with your friends and catch up with old
friends you might have lost touch with

Remember Self-Compassion

Becoming mindful of the emotions you experience throughout the day,
without judging yourself, builds your self-compassion. Self-compassion can
start with trying to talk to yourself as kindly as you would speak to a friend
or loved one.

The more we practice self-compassion, the better we become at taking
care of ourselves. The better able we are to take care of ourselves, the more
we are able to take care of others. It might seem silly, but having a positive mantra to say when you are feeling especially negative about yourself
can be helpful. The next time you catch yourself beating yourself up over
something, repeat one of these statements three times: "I am strong." "I am
going to be okay." "I am enough." This is especially important when you
feel your illness encroaching on your "normal" life. Extend the compassion
to yourself that you do to others.

Work to Find the Good in the World

One of the major contributors to chronic activation of stress is our own
worldview. More important than income or education, people who view
their social world as hostile, unsupportive, and threatening are more likely
to have more significant inflammatory responses to stress than those who
believe that they benefit from their social connections. It is not the number
of friends you have or your marital status that affects the level of inflammation you experience from stress, but your own belief about your social support network. With the help of a therapist, workbooks, lifestyle changes, or
medical treatment of depression, you can start to reframe how you see the
world. We know it sounds easy to say this, but as with everything else, we
recommend small changes.

Invest Time in Improving Your Breathing

We all breathe about ten to twelve times a minute. When we are stressed, our breathing rate can increase as our heart rate increases. Deep relaxation breathing or even sharp inhales through the nostrils can trigger your parasympathetic nervous system, your body's calming response. Just as your brain can control your lungs, going fast when you're scared, you can control your lungs so that they tell your brain it's time to chill.

Spend Time in Nature

Being in nature makes us feel good. Time spent in green spaces not only reduces stress but improves sleep, attention, creativity, memory, and athletic performance, makes us happy, and has other benefits as well. The natural world improves your health by absorbing pollutants, reducing sound pollution, and increasing neighborhood cohesiveness, which can increase socializing and decrease loneliness.

Here are some ways to increase your "green time" to turn down stress:

Add some plants inside your home, or grow some seeds in a pot on your porch.

Join a local community garden. While cultivating your own garden plot or helping others tend to theirs, you can meet neighbors and sometimes get free fruit, vegetables, and plants.

Encourage gardening in your community's schools and parks.

Look on a map to locate the parks and nature areas near your home and make plans to visit them. Some have outdoor exercise equipment that anyone can use.

If you bike, look for bike trails that take you through parks or on nature routes.

Spend time with animals: take a dog on a walk, roam the neighborhood with a cat, watch birds fly around your street.

Take exercise classes outdoors. Bring your phone and play a workout
   video or meditation surrounded by trees or in a public garden.

Play nature sounds in your house.

Grab a Frisbee, bubbles, or a ball and play outside with your kids, your
   neighbors, or your friends.

Go to a beach, pond, or lake and take a walk. Get in the water if the
   conditions are right.

If you find yourself in nature, pause, take a deep breath, and enjoy the
   beauty.

EXERCISE

BREATHE WITH A TREE

Trees remove carbon dioxide and pollutants from the air and release oxygen. They are beautiful to look at and provide us with a sense of calmness.

   Find a tree near your home, even if you have to travel a little bit. (If you
can't get to a tree, look online.) Go sit next to the tree. Take three slow
deep breaths, in and out. Notice the trunk of the tree and the roots running underground beneath you. Feel the strength of the roots supporting
you and holding you up.

   If you feel comfortable and your body will allow you to do so, lie down
and look up the trunk of the tree into the branches. As you continue
with slow deep breaths, watch or feel the branches and leaves move in
the breeze. Even on a windless day, the tree still appears to be moving,
or breathing. Breathe with the tree, inhaling deep into your nose and fill-
ing your lungs, then slowly breathing out. Practice this for five minutes or
more.

   If you want to continue this meditation, think about the life of the tree.
It started out as a little seed and then grew over many years to this giant
living creature. It is amazing that it is helping you stay alive by giving you
oxygen to breathe.

Your Stress Response and Resilience

How is it that some people are susceptible to stressors and others are more resilient? Your response to stress is encoded in your DNA; inherited factors determine your capacity for resilience. Your stress response is also subject to epigenetic factors: environmental factors that affect your gene expression. These genetic differences make some people more susceptible to the effects of stress. Because they have stronger inflammatory responses to adversity, they are at higher risk of inflammatory-related disease.

Experiences early in life can turn on different epigenetic pathways that affect gene expression and affect how we react to stress in the future. Some early events coach us in resilience and build up our tolerance of stress. Stress resilience training helps us tap into our coping mechanisms more quickly, and as with physical exercise, using coping skills helps us feel better faster, making us more likely to use them more often and more quickly. We all can improve and get better at resilience, regardless of our genetic makeup or adverse experiences. There are many resources that can help you by simulating stressful situations to help build your resilience, practice coping skills, and increase your insight into how you handle stress, including apps, websites, practitioners, and support groups.

Let's return to the U-shaped curve in the figure on page 216. Being able to cope with a moderate amount of stress can make you feel like you can handle that level of stress. That feeling promotes your resilience in future encounters with stress. Maintaining optimal stress exposure is protective, as we all are going to encounter stressors at some point. Many experiments have shown that enhancing stress tolerance early in life promotes resilience later on. Even if you have a genetic predisposition to a strong inflammatory reaction to stress, you can still stack the odds in your favor.

Note: The concept of stress resilience has been co-opted by employers and others as a characteristic to look for in potential employees or as marks of a strong person. When people talk about resilience with you, make sure the intention is to make your life easier and better. The goal of increasing your resilience is not to enable you to deal with terrible people at work, put up with unfair policies, and accept low wages. The goal of increasing your resilience is to make you feel better and more capable of dealing with unexpected life situations. Be wary of those who tell you that a certain experience or job will give you more grit or resilience. You get enough of that from your long illness and from life as it is. For more on resilience, see Chapter 22.

EXERCISE

UNSIGN UP

One of the most important lessons you can learn in long illness is how to protect your time. Many of us underestimate how stressed out we might become when we take on too much. The more stress you have, the more likely you are to have a flare-up. If you feel stressed about having enough time to do things for yourself, or as though you have too much to do in a certain area of your life, there are many helpful tools you can use, including to-do lists, family meetings, therapy, and delegating tasks. If you have a job, your workplace may offer training to improve your resilience and coping skills, though most of these trainings are aimed at being more productive for someone else.

Let's try this exercise:

- Look at your schedule and to-do list for this week. Put a check mark next to everything you are excited about doing. These are what you are going to do this week.
- Look at the items on your list you didn't check. Sure, you can't say no to all of them. But look at them again:
  - Can someone else take one of these tasks?
  - Can you reschedule or skip meetings?
- Can you move some appointments to virtual to cut down on travel? Most importantly, which items on your to-do list did you agree to do that you didn't really want to do in the first place? What has turned into something you no longer want to do?

Here is a script to use to unsign up over the phone, in person, or by text or email:

> *Hello, [name]. I have enjoyed the time I have spent on [activity or responsibility]. However, for the next few weeks (months), I am going to be taking a break.*

Or:

> *However, now is a good time for me to step away.*

Or:

> *However, I cannot take on additional responsibilities at this time. I look forward to working with you again in the future. In appreciation, [your name]*

Here is how to say "no" *before* signing up:

> *That sounds interesting (fun/exciting/cool). I would love to be involved, but I am going to have to say no to this one. Good luck and let me know how it turns out.*

Or:

> *No, I can't right now.*

Or:

> *No, I can't.*

Or:

> *No.*

"No" is a complete sentence.

You don't need to say "sorry." You do not need to give reasons. You can set a simple boundary and just say "no." It doesn't mean you don't care.

Setting a boundary may make you feel anxious or guilty. Those feelings are something to reflect on. Your stress level directly impacts your health. And your health needs to be a priority in long illness. You can practice saying "no" if you know you are going to be in a situation where you will be asked to contribute and you simply cannot. If you don't feel comfortable with setting boundaries, working with a therapist or friend to learn how to do so comfortably is a good place to start.

EXERCISE

JOURNAL YOUR STRESS

Think of a recent time you experienced a minor stressful event.

What happened?

How did your body feel?

What emotions were you feeling?

How did you react?

Did you talk to anyone about what happened? How did that change your perception of the situation?

If you were in the situation again, would you do anything differently?

CHAPTER 17

Fueling Your Body Through Long Illness

You have to eat. Food is not optional. There is so much information, sometimes conflicting, and always overwhelming. When to eat, what to eat, how to prepare it, and to be honest, I don't believe there is a right way for anyone to eat, it changes day to day. Which is what makes it hard. Over time, with lots of trial and error, I have figured out some things that work for my body. I am always fine-tuning it, trying new things, and always learning more. But most of the time I just stick to what is simple and what decreases my symptoms. It took me years to learn how to do this, but I try to pay attention to how I feel after I eat, in the hours and days. I feel physically the best when I eat an anti-inflammatory diet, but I am human. I make sure I allow for the joys that food can bring. I try to look at the big picture and have compassion for cravings. I give myself leeway for the things that bring me joy and have learned ways to keep all the foods that I love. It's still hard. Just be patient with yourself as you try to learn what is best for your body.

What's the best fuel for my body?" "How can nutrition change my health?" These are important questions in long illness, especially if your body is already dealing with inflammation and stress. Although ordinarily a plant-rich, anti-inflammatory diet gives us the vitamins and minerals we need, people with long illness can have suboptimal levels of vitamins and minerals.

Optimizing your nutrition can shift the health of your cells, organs, joints, and skin. This chapter will help you work with your health care team to assess your nutritional status and consume foods that support healing and prevent flares and relapse. We separate nutrition and food here because nutrition, in our definition, is the nuts-and-bolts science of food and how it relates to disease.

Before we dive in, we want to acknowledge that some long illnesses make eating and issues around food uncomfortable. For example, if you have gastrointestinal disease, you may associate eating with pain. If you have an eating disorder or another condition that requires specific attention to food, such as diabetes, you may have questions and feel unable to nourish yourself. Working with a team of practitioners who consider your nutritional, gastrointestinal, and psychological needs is helpful as you try to return to healthy eating patterns. As with all other advice in this book, what we say here about nutrition is not meant to add more stress to your life.

What You Will Learn in This Chapter:

- Why the content of your food matters in long illness
- How metabolism and inflammation are connected
- How to track your food intake to see if you are meeting your nutritional needs

Nutrition 101

When we eat food, it's broken down by our digestive tract into molecules called *macronutrients*, which are nutrients we need in large (macro) amounts. Macronutrients provide energy, form the body, and regulate chemical processes in the body. The ones you are probably most familiar with are carbohydrates, fats, and protein.

Carbohydrates are simple sugars that can be rapidly turned into energy in the form of glucose. You might have heard people talk about simple and complex carbs. They are referring to how long it takes to turn food into glucose. Faster is not better. Excess glucose is stored as fat in the liver and elsewhere in the body.

Carbs have gotten a bad rap, but not all carbs are created equal. Minimally processed grains (steel-cut oats instead of instant flavored oatmeal, for instance), vegetables, fruits, and beans are all good sources of carbs. Generally, you should avoid highly processed and refined foods in order to reduce inflammation and protect your brain health. Limit yummy pastries, cake, soda, and white bread to special occasions, as eating them regularly can increase inflammation.

Fats store energy and support cellular health. In the 1980s, fats were unfairly vilified, and that reputation has stuck despite decades of good science proving otherwise. Unsaturated fats, which keep your nervous and immune systems healthy, include omega-3 fatty acids. Many diets are low in omega-3 fatty acids, so chances are yours is too. Omega-3 fatty acids are found in fatty fish, nuts, flaxseed, soy, and avocados. Usually 30 percent of your calories should come from healthy fats. Limit your consumption of saturated fats, since they do not provide a health benefit.

Protein is made up of amino acids, many of which your body gets from food. (It also makes amino acids.) If you don't eat enough protein, your body will start breaking down muscle to get amino acids, which it needs for almost everything. Protein is found not just in meat but can come from many sources, including nuts, dairy, eggs, and plants. Calories from protein should make up about 30 percent of your daily intake.

Micronutrients, Macrominerals, and Trace Minerals

Vitamins and minerals are also nutrients. They are called *micronutrients* because your body needs them in small amounts (less than 100 milligrams a day) to function. Vitamins and minerals are carried throughout your body in fat (fat-soluble vitamins) or water (water-soluble vitamins). Similarly, trace minerals are needed in very small amounts (in micrograms), and macrominerals are needed in relatively larger amounts (in grams). True deficiencies in vitamins and minerals can result in serious medical conditions and death. Most people in industrialized countries who eat a standard diet are getting some amount of most vitamins and minerals because many processed foods have been enriched with added vitamins and minerals. As a result, severe deficiencies are less common. (See the tables in Appendix E for information on micronutrients, macronutrients, and trace minerals.)

Long illness, however, can leave you vulnerable to deficiencies by affecting your food choices, tolerance, absorption, and need for certain nutrients. Taking handfuls of supplements every day is not the best way to address these deficiencies. Eating food is how our bodies have evolved to absorb nutrients, so optimizing your diet is the best way to improve your nutrition. This said, you might want to assess your diet for how much it supplies some nutrients that are commonly low in many people.

What Nutrients Could You Be Missing in Your Diet?

Worldwide, and especially in the United States, diets are low in vitamin D, calcium, and fiber. Insufficient hydration is another concern. Let's explore these often-missing nutrients needed for the body to thrive.

Vitamin D

Vitamin D helps your gut absorb calcium. It also reduces inflammation, helps your bones and muscles function and grow, helps with sleep, brain health, and mood regulation, and plays a role in energy metabolism. You get vitamin D from the sun; if you have darker skin, you need more sun to make the same amount of vitamin D a lighter-skinned person gets. "Go outside for fifteen minutes daily" is not sufficient advice for maintaining adequate vitamin D levels for most of us; we just don't spend enough time outside. Not to mention that the sun might not be out regularly where you live, and sunlight can cause burns, overheating, and skin cancer. Few foods contain vitamin D naturally, which is why in some countries milk and milk alternatives are fortified with vitamin D. Oily fishes have the highest amounts; vitamin D is also available in red meat, liver, egg yolks, and mushrooms.

Guidelines for how much vitamin D you need can vary, which is why some of you may have been told you have normal vitamin D and others with the same number are told that their number is low. For many people, we recommend supplementing vitamin D to get your blood level above 30 ng/mL (nanograms per milliliter) (75 nmol/L [nanomoles per liter]) with 1,000–2,000 IU (international units) daily—but no higher than 50–60 ng/mL, as that is when side effects might begin to occur. Severe deficiency is uniformly treated with high vitamin D supplementation for a few weeks, after which levels are retested. You should not be on a supplement higher than 2,000 IU daily for an extended period of time unless your practitioner specifically recommends it. Sometimes a once-a-month supplement can be taken to reduce the number of pills taken in a day.

Vitamin D deficiency is more common in people with dark skin, and it increases with age, a vegetarian or vegan diet, limited sun exposure, or fat malabsorption (which can occur with GI diseases and cystic fibrosis and after gastric surgery). An active area of research is looking at the lower levels of vitamin D in people with various health conditions. It is unclear if low vitamin D contributes to the development of autoimmune illnesses or is associated with those illnesses for other reasons. However, low vitamin D does seem to precede the development of several autoimmune diseases. There is hope that supplementation with vitamin D can reduce the risk of autoimmune disease or change its course. And of course, for those of you who are on steroid medication or have thinning of the bones for other reasons (osteopenia, osteoporosis), the recommendation is to be on a combination of vitamin D and calcium.

Calcium

Calcium is an elemental metal that plays many roles in your body. Calcium helps make your bones and blood cells and is essential for digestion, circulation, and physical activity.

Women tend to get less calcium in their diets. Also, women who are postmenopausal or do not have periods do not have adequate estrogen levels to support a healthy calcium blood level. Also at risk are vegetarians and young women between nineteen and thirty (whose bones are still growing).

Foods rich in calcium include dairy products, greens (kale, collards, spinach, broccoli), eggs, beans, lentils, nuts, seeds, and soy. Many multivitamin and mineral supplements contain some calcium, but only small amounts.

We generally recommend that young women and menopausal women ensure that they get adequate calcium and vitamin D in their diet through food. If your calcium intake is consistently low through food, despite your efforts, or you have absorption issues, we recommend supplementation under the guidance of a practitioner who is aware of your risk factors and needs.

Fiber

There are two types of fiber, soluble and insoluble. Fiber is a sugar (carbohydrate) in plant-based foods that is difficult for your body to absorb or digest. It gives bulk to your gut contents, helps your intestines contract to move the food along, slows down food movement so that nutrients can be absorbed, slows increases in blood sugar levels, and provides food for your microbiome (see Chapter 9 on gut health). People who eat diets high in fiber have lower cholesterol, lower blood pressure, less heart disease, and a healthier weight.

We estimate that one out of ten of you reading this gets enough fiber in your diet. You read that correctly—one out of ten! Only 15 percent of people in the United States eat enough vegetables, fruits, and whole grains, the sources of most fiber. Beans, leafy greens, whole grains, and orange vegetables have the highest fiber content. Fiber-enriched cereals are also a good way to boost fiber consumption. Adding high-fiber foods to each meal in small amounts is the best way to increase fiber. If you increase your fiber quickly, you could experience gas, bloating, and other intestinal upset.

WHEN LOW-FIBER DIETS ARE HELPFUL

Low-fiber diets are recommended for those undergoing some chemotherapy and radiation treatments. After the gut has healed, fiber can be slowly added back by eating foods that you tolerate best. Sometimes a low-fiber diet is recommended—most commonly for people who are having an episode of inflammatory bowel disease or gastroparesis—when there has been damage to the gut. For those with gastrointestinal disease, eating can be painful, so working with a team of practitioners who consider your nutritional, gastrointestinal, and psychological needs can be helpful.

Water

As covered in Chapter 15, water should be the primary beverage you drink. Staying hydrated protects your kidneys from stones and urinary tract infections, improves your skin elasticity, prevents constipation, protects your brain and spinal cord, lubricates and cushions your joints, cools you down when you exert yourself, and helps you excrete waste products through sweat, urine, and bowel movements. Poor hydration can lead to headaches, mental fog, decreased athletic and cognitive performance, agitation, poor sleep quality, lower energy, overeating, low mood, and more.

The Institute of Medicine recommends that the average person drink nine to thirteen cups of water a day in addition to the two to three cups most of us get from our diet. People who are larger, who exercise, or who are on certain medications, like antihistamines and some antidepressants, need more water. An easy way to know if you are drinking enough? Look at your urine. If it is dark, drink more water. The goal is light yellow urine, but not clear.

EXERCISE

WATER SWAP

Tomorrow swap all your beverages (aside from one to two cups of black coffee or plain tea if you need it) to water. During the day, think about times when you drink beverages that are not water. What are you drinking? Are there any swaps you could make? Did you feel any different after switching to all water for the day?

Other Important Nutrients

Magnesium, potassium, iron, choline, and vitamins A, C, D, and E are underconsumed by most Americans. Additionally, zinc and B_{12} levels could be low in vegetarians. Take a look at the tables in Appendix E on page 326. Are you eating some of the foods listed there that are rich in these nutrients? Can you add two or three of these foods to your plate each week?

Do You Need a Multivitamin and Mineral Pill?

As we note at the start of this chapter, people with long illness can have sub-optimal levels of vitamins and minerals owing to poor absorption, limited dietary intake, inability to tolerate varied diets, or lack of access to nourishing food. There isn't enough evidence that taking a multivitamin and mineral (MVM) supplement daily will prevent disease or help you live longer, but we recommend MVM pills for patients with chronic illness, especially during times of illness, stress, or inadequate diet. People who take MVM supplements are more likely to meet their requirements for daily nutrients compared to those who do not. Your aim should be to get 100 percent of your daily recommended value of nutrients. With vitamins and minerals, more is not necessarily better, so aim for an MVM that only supplements your needs, not one that completely replaces it. As always, you should check with your practitioner before you begin taking any supplements.

What Are You Eating Too Much Of?

Salt, sugar, and saturated fats are pro-inflammatory foods. They are often tasty, but only salt is actually needed by your body. Consumed once in a while, a small amount of sugar, saturated fats, or alcohol is probably not a big deal. But if you are already sick and stressed, we suggest that you pause before adding fuel to the fire.

Salt. Salt is high in processed foods, where most of our sodium intake comes from. Cutting down on processed foods is a great way to decrease your sodium intake. Diets high in sodium put you at greater risk of developing high blood pressure, which increases your risk of stroke and heart disease. On an average day, an American will eat 3,400 milligrams of sodium, which is much higher than the recommended 2,300 milligrams. The American Heart Association sets the ideal limit at no more than 1,500 milligrams of sodium a day, as your body needs only 500 milligrams daily to function. Dropping to 1,500 milligrams is recommended for everyone, with the exception of those with heart failure, people who sweat significant amounts (athletes, firefighters), and those with less common health conditions. Talk to your practitioners about the sodium level goal that's right for your health needs.

Sugar. The average American eats 300–400 calories a day in sugar (about 20–24 teaspoons). Don't feel like that is possible? Sugar hides in many foods. It is added to many prepared foods, like soups and breads, to enhance the flavor, and sugar also shows up in sauces, condiments, and dressings. Most of us underestimate the amount of sugar we put in our bodies. It all adds up: soft drinks, fruit drinks, flavored yogurt, cookies, pastries, candy, most processed foods—it's too much. Diets higher in added sugar can lead to diabetes, obesity, heart disease, high blood pressure, chronic inflammation, fatty liver disease, cognitive impairment, and more.

There are many easy ways to cut down on sugar. Scaling back on processed foods, drinking only water, black coffee, and plain tea, and saying no to unplanned sweets are simple ways to lessen your sugar intake. It is recommended that no more than 10 percent of your daily calories come from sugar, which is equal to one can of soda.

Saturated fats. Saturated fats occur naturally in many foods, including red meat, whole dairy products, cheese, and coconut oil. Many processed foods are high in saturated fats, as well as salt and added sugars, so cutting down on them can have multiple benefits. Diets high in saturated fats increase total cholesterol and decrease healthy fats.

Replacing saturated fats with heart-protective polyunsaturated fats (olive oil) or high-fiber carbohydrates (beans, vegetables) can reduce the risk of heart disease. For those who favor coconut oil, there isn't great data, but if you eat a generally healthy diet, coconut oil in moderation is okay.

What Exactly Is Processed Food?

Over the last few generations, we have seen minimally processed foods and meals prepared at home replaced with fast foods and ultra-processed foods. Food science has had many positive effects on human health, but the processing of food has gone from helpful to harmful. New research aimed at classifying how much a food is processed has found that it's not just the ingredients but how they are processed and modified that is making these foods pro-inflammatory.

Processing at some level is necessary in an industrialized society. Not everyone is a farmer, and not everyone can afford fresh food daily. Food has to be transported, prepared, and stored for the many people who live in cities. Many of our foods are at least minimally processed. However, *ultra-processing* has dialed processing up a notch. Many of the processing techniques used today cannot be used at home unless you live in a laboratory. Whole foods are broken down into their constituent parts, modified, re-formed into new foodlike substances, filled with additives and preservatives, and put in an irresistible shiny package on shelves halfway around the world. Most of the ingredients in ultra-processed food are substances you have never seen on your pantry shelf and additives that make it edible, such as emulsifiers, sweeteners, thickeners, flavors, and colors. Research indicates that additives and preservatives are inflammatory and harmful to human health. Increased consumption of ultra-processed foods is associated with a higher risk of cardiovascular and cerebrovascular disease and an increased risk of cancer, diabetes, obesity, irritable bowel syndrome, and more.

Most ultra-processed food is low in fiber and natural compounds but full of calories, salt, sugar, and saturated (trans) fats. Since our complex bodies run on nutrients and can clean up only a finite amount of toxins and chemicals, ultra-processed foods are a real threat to our well-being.

Advertising for many ultra-processed foods claims they are healthy because they have added chemical nutrients like vitamins and fiber or have had salt removed. Don't be fooled. The food-processing companies pay big bucks to advertise these unhealthy foods to you in ways that make them hard for you to resist. The fact that these foods are often less expensive than unprocessed food and can be easier to access than healthy foods adds another layer to the discussion: if your illness has affected your income, you may not have access to food that can help you feel better. Your finances shouldn't exclude you from being able to get the medicine through food that your body needs to reduce inflammation and have more energy.

This is not all on you. There are many obstacles to consistently accessing and eating healthy foods. Although you might not be able to eat a perfect healthy plate of food at each meal, you *can* eat a healthier meal. We'll talk more about this in the next chapter.

What Is Metabolic Flexibility?

When we talk about nutrition, it is useful to talk about metabolism and how it relates to long illness. Your body switches between the different types of fuels that you take in based on your overall state of health. This type of metabolic regulation was essential for survival in times of feast and famine, but it poses a problem in the era of food delivery apps.

Your body uses two types of fuel to make energy: fat and sugar. When your glucose levels are low because you have been exercising or haven't eaten for a long time, your body uses fat to get energy. Fat is a great energy source. The problem is that your brain prefers to run on sugar and doesn't use fat very well. During times of stress, other tissues will use fat and let the brain use glucose (sugar) for energy.

Imagine eating a big meal, then ordering takeout from all of your favorite places. Everything arrives at the same time. Imagine how you would feel. This is how the average Western diet makes your mitochondria feel.

This overwhelmed feeling results in *metabolic inflexibility*—your body's inability to use all of its fuel sources. Metabolic inflexibility has been found in numerous chronic and long illnesses. When your body is unable to use energy quickly, your metabolism is off, which can lead to issues like brain fog, fatigue, confusion, and memory lapses. Metabolic inflexibility also leads to insulin resistance throughout your body, putting you at risk of developing diabetes and other diseases. No medication currently on the market or in development is better for improving your body's metabolic flexibility than an optimized diet and regular movement.

What Does Metabolism Have to Do with Inflammation?

Metabolism provides the energy source for chronic inflammation. As noted earlier, many cells in your body release chemicals, called cytokines (or adipokines in fat), that generally increase inflammation. The immune system tries to help but often releases more inflammation signals when it kicks in.

It's a song on repeat. You're stuck in a loop. Signals from a sick, overworked system increase inflammation and cause your immune system to attack your own tissue (*autoimmunity*). While this is happening in one part of your body, your brain is keeping tabs and responds to inflammation like it is an emergency. This response amplifies the stress signal and increases inflammation. For your body, stress is loaded upon stress.

The extra energy is then stored as fat cells, which, in excess, can release more inflammatory signals. Initially, this signal turns up your metabolism so that you burn more calories from fat. As fat accumulates over time, however, your body starts to respond less to the signals from the cells. Your metabolism slows down because it no longer responds well to the signals from your cells. This is one of the many reasons it can be hard to lose weight when you have a long illness. Increased inflammation can also lead to insulin resistance, which can lead to a host of problems that slow down and impact metabolism and inflammation. Metabolism can be supported by strengthening and movement, intermittent fasting, and anti-inflammatory diets.

Journaling

SO WHAT *ARE* YOU EATING?

The goal of this exercise is to record and review what you are putting into your body. If you are not in a place to do this, come back and visit this exercise when you are. *For some of you, tracking your food can be triggering, so stop and skip to the next section.* The purpose of this exercise is for you to observe the nutritional content of your intake, not judge your intake. If you see where you might be able to make a nutritious change, then we support you in trying that. Our goal is to support you in fueling your body, especially if your body is already dealing with impacts from long illness. For those of you who haven't taken stock of what you are putting into your body lately, step back and take a look.

FOOD TRACKING

Tracking what you eat and drink will give you information to compare to the information in some of the charts and tables in this book and an opportunity to reflect on what you are eating and drinking. You can use pen and paper to keep track or, if you have internet access, one of the many apps that are aimed at different nutritional goals, including tracking nutrient intake. Most apps calculate macronutrients for free. Sadly, we've been unable to find a free app that calculates micronutrients simply and is easy to use.

If you have used an app that you like, feel free to use it for this exercise. If not, you can start with the US Department of Agriculture's "Start Simple with MyPlate" app. With this app you can track your food group intake daily. It is a good place to start if you are new to food tracking or don't want to enter foods or get distracted with calories and too much other information. Nutritional recommendations fluctuate and vary for different conditions, but none of the recommendations are written in stone. The app makes "Dietary Guidelines for Americans for 2020 to 2025" available for free, and its many tools are useful for both people with minimal nutritional knowledge and those with more nutritional knowledge.

For this exercise, go to the "Start Simple with MyPlate" app (www.myplate.gov/tip-sheet/start-simple-myplate) to get access to the

MyPlate quiz. Once you have entered your findings for a few days, look at the data you have collected. Look over the different sections of this chapter. How are you doing with nutrient intake? What nutrients could you eat more of? Are there nutrients you are eating too much of? What about your intake of sugar, saturated fats, and salt?

Write down three things that you are proud of about your food tracking.

Write down at least one thing you can do differently today to improve your nutrition.

Visit your food journal every two weeks and consider doing the exercise again after you have made a few changes. In our next chapter, we will talk about dietary eating patterns, or what you eat over time. Hopefully some of those diets will give you an idea of some themes you can try to incorporate into your eating habits to improve your overall nutrition and health.

Sample Food Diary

Diaries or journals to track habits are pretty similar. The goal is to record information about what you are doing so that you can go back and reflect on your activities later. In a food diary, you can look for triggers by tracking symptoms (we talk more about sensitivities and elimination diets in Chapter 18), track your intake of macronutrients and micronutrients, and get a sense of your overall dietary trends, like noting those times when you made less positive food choices. Keeping a food journal is a good choice if you have food allergies or gastrointestinal issues because it can help you identify foods that are worsening your symptoms.

Although we love this tool, it is not for everyone. If you have a history of an eating disorder, we recommend discussing a food diary with your team before exploring this tool further.

When setting up a food journal, start with as many or as few variables as you like, and modify it in the way that works best for you. It is easier to keep it simple at first for a few days, focusing on what you are interested in. To get a picture of your general intake, eat how you regularly eat for a few days and write down everything that goes into your mouth. Here are some examples:

FOOD DIARY: EXAMPLE 1

Time	What I Ate	Where	Thoughts/Feelings
6:00 a.m.	Frosted flakes, banana, skim milk, orange juice, coffee	Home	Big burst of energy, hungry when I woke up, ate 5 minutes after I woke up
1:00 p.m.	Salad, grilled chicken, ranch dressing, Diet Coke, baked potato chips	Work	Starving, headache before eating, ate fast at the computer, still felt hungry after eating
3:00 p.m.	Caramel skim milk latte, pumpkin chocolate chip bread	Work	Hungry after lunch, felt tired like I needed a pick-me-up, crashed about an hour later
7:00 p.m.	Fried chicken, mashed potatoes, gravy, carrots, biscuit, cherry pie, iced tea	Restaurant	Ate too much with friends, stomach hurt
10:00 p.m.	Popcorn with butter, handful of M&M's	Home	Wanted snack to wind me down before bed, stomach felt full, ate watching TV, hard to fall asleep

There are different ways to evaluate a diary.

Taking it in: For some, just seeing what they eat in a day can be revealing. Many of us underestimate how much we eat and overestimate how healthy the food we eat is.

Nutrient check: You can track nutrients on an app that calculates your nutrient intake based on what you eat. For instance, the food log here shows that this person ate 3,329 calories, 126 grams of fat (35 unsaturated), 429 grams of carbs, 129 grams of protein, 5,833 grams of sodium, 32 grams of fiber, and 112 grams of sugar.[6]

Trends: This food log shows that this person had caffeine four times in a day, let a long time elapse between breakfast and lunch, ate most of their calories later in the day, and ate sweets multiple times.

Thoughts and feelings: The food log states a lack of satisfaction from the food consumed. This person felt hungry despite the high number of calories they ate, food affected their sleep, and food seemed connected to highs and lows in mood and energy they experienced throughout the day.

What else do you see? Do you have any suggestions for how to improve this person's diet?

FOOD DIARY: EXAMPLE 2

Time	What I Ate	Where	Thoughts/Feelings
8:00 a.m.	2 scrambled eggs, 1/2 avocado, 2 pieces whole-grain toast, olive oil	Home	Ate slowly
12:00 p.m.	Tuna salad in pita with lettuce, handful of baby carrots, cherry tomatoes	Work	Got hungry at 11:45, ate slowly outside while not checking email, felt full after
3:00 p.m.	Tablespoon peanut butter, celery	Work	Ate my snack because it was 3:00 p.m. Went on a walk around the building after.
7:00 p.m.	Lentils, brown rice, roasted cauliflower in olive oil	Home	Felt full, and that I could have had less, but dinner was so tasty. Ate at the table with family, no TV.

Taking it in: This diet is nutritious and diverse.

Nutrient check: This person ate 1,737 calories, 70 grams of fat (16 unsaturated), 165 grams of carbs, 104 grams of protein, 1,982 grams of sodium, 43 grams of fiber, and 26 grams of sugar.

Trends: This log shows many different types of vegetables, healthy fats, and antioxidants.

Thoughts and feelings: This person ate slowly, ate despite not being hungry and was aware of this, and had hunger cues close to when it was time to eat.

What else do you see? Do you have any suggestions for how to improve this person's diet?

This food log may look healthier than the first one, but there are tips and tricks for optimizing almost any diet. For example, if this person is not used to eating this much fiber and certain fruits and vegetables, they might be having gas. It is good to also note physical responses in a food log.

Questions for Your Medical Team

Most practitioners will begin by having you track your food, so be one step ahead and keep a food diary for three to five days to get a sense of what you are eating. Keep in mind that not all practitioners have the knowledge to talk with you about your nutritional needs, but they should be able to review your intake with you, make suggestions, and point you toward others who can be more helpful.

Based on my condition, should I have a nutritionist or dietitian on my team?

If you have insurance, ask what is covered by your plan. Some primary care clinics have embedded nutrition and dietary support, especially for those with certain conditions.

Based on my condition, are there any nutrients I might be deficient in? Should I be regularly testing for any of these nutrients? Should I be taking something regularly based on my condition, or can I try to get it from food?

While most healthcare practitioners don't have a lot of training in nutrition, they may be able to tell you basic deficiencies (such as vitamin D, B vitamins); as above, they may also be able to refer you to a nutritionist.

Am I eligible for medically tailored meals (for example, a renal diet, or a diabetic diet), medically tailored groceries, produce prescriptions, or other nutritionally based programs?

Some primary care clinics can help patients access various programs that help you get free or reduced-cost foods. Some even deliver.

When I was in college, I got really sick and found out I was eligible for a food delivery program through my student meal plan. Each week, a bag of healthy groceries were delivered to me. It really helped having the "safe food" that wouldn't make me sick like the pizza station and cereal bar at the cafeteria. When I was feeling better, myself and other students who had used the program helped to make the cafeterias healthier and we were able to stock the student stores with healthy snacks. While it was hard to pick almonds over ice cream, at least there was an option.

EXERCISE

MINDFUL BITE

Connecting more deeply to the nutrition within food is an opportunity to cultivate mindfulness. Try this simple exercise to begin slowing down and appreciating all the dimensions of food.

Grab a slice of fruit, a handful of nuts, or a piece of dark chocolate.

Sight: *Look at the food. What is its shape and color?*

Touch: *What does the food feel like in your hand? Is it rough or smooth? Is it heavy or light?*

Smell: *Bring the food up to your nose and appreciate the smell. What does it smell like? Is it a strong odor or a mild one? Does it bring any memories to mind?*

Taste: *Put the food on your tongue, but do not chew it yet. What does it taste like?*

Bite: *Begin to bite down and slowly chew the food. Has the taste changed?*

Reflect: *What was this experience like? Is this food nutritious and good for your body?*

Many people find that even just a single mindful bite with each meal connects them more deeply with their food. It allows them to slow down and sense the feeling of fullness more quickly and to experience food in a richer way.

Mindful eating is a practice. Refer to our resources section to learn more about mindful eating skills on trusted websites.

CHAPTER 18

Enjoy Food, Nourish Yourself

When I eat an anti-inflammatory diet 100 percent of the time, I feel the best. Honestly, I don't eat like that all the time. I think it's important to find what works for your body, but also give it some leeway to enjoy things that bring you joy from eating. I have found that despite all my allergies, really strict diets are so prohibitive they can limit my enjoyment of food. I think that a little bit of grace is needed in diet and nutrition. Look at the big picture. It's not what you eat for a day or a week. It's over long stretches.

What You Will Learn in This Chapter:

- The compelling reasons to optimize and find the right diet for your long illness
- An overview of the science and medicine behind the most common diets used in long illness: Mediterranean, vegetarian, DASH, intermittent fasting, and low-carb
- An exploration of diets that target specific health complaints, such as the elimination diet, the autoimmune protocol diet, the FODMaP diet, and the MIND diet
- Ways to reduce free radical exposure by increasing antioxidants in your diet
- Tips for shifting your diet in a balanced, realistic way

Having a long illness is hard. With so many things to juggle in a time of crisis, it's no surprise if you fall back on old habits. Our hope with this chapter is to provide you with evidence-based information on the most common ways of eating that can be helpful to incorporate into your long illness recovery. Certain ways of eating might be helpful while your body is inflamed and in repair mode, especially during flare-ups. People living with illness and disability often must pay more attention to what they eat to make sure they get the nutrients they need and to avoid inflammatory foods that might worsen their underlying condition.

First, a note about word choice: "diet" is a troubling word for many people. It is often associated with restriction, decreased pleasure, and unrealistic body expectations. We use the word "diet" here, however, in its most general sense—simply to refer to the kind of food that you regularly eat. You'll notice that we talk about "healthy eating patterns" throughout. Whatever words we use, know that we intend to broaden the scope rather than focus on trendy, problematic "diets."

The purpose of educating yourself about different foods you might want to restrict or remove from your diet is not to create an unhealthy relationship with certain foods. Nothing about diet is black and white. The best way of eating for you may not be the best for someone else. In the future, personalized nutrition based on gut microbiome, genetics, metabolic profiles, and your environment will be available. For now, we have solid data that give a good basic understanding of what people should be eating. Determining what specifically works for you will be trial and error. And what works for you now might change over time. Be patient with yourself. Reducing or eliminating some foods might be better for your symptoms and your health. However, we usually recommend trying to add them back later.

Why Improve Your Diet?

Much diet advice is too focused on weight loss. This is not helpful for many reasons. We want you to refocus your dietary goals on supporting your vitality. This often means targeting *fat loss* or *muscle gain*. Why? Fat cells (adipose cells) are pro-inflammatory. Muscle cells (myocytes) are anti-inflammatory. Even losing a bit of body fat—and, even better, replacing it with some muscle mass—*can change how your body feels and performs.*

When you feel better, it's easier to accept your body and its shape, size, or scars. With many of your friends who don't have long illness trying out fad diets, you might think that a quick fix will point you in the right direction. But there are no shortcuts or magic tricks here. While it's okay to try different ways of eating, it's important to remember that your needs might be different than those of a friend who can tolerate more restrictive, stressful, or pro-inflammatory diets.

A healthy diet is simple, but it isn't easy. We are wired to eat, but many of us have been wired to eat unhealthy foods and in unhealthy quantities. Unlearning habits takes time, reeducation, and self-compassion. Slowly, but surely, you can make better decisions about your nutrition. If you notice that your habits are difficult to understand, or that you are obsessing on or overthinking your dietary choices, consider mentioning this to your care team to see if additional support from a therapist or other resources might be helpful.

Even when we learn about new ways of eating, it can be hard to make sustainable shifts. In this chapter, we give you tools to make small changes toward a diet that is aligned with your health goals. Like many things in long illness recovery, we aim for progress, not perfection.

If you read this chapter and get overwhelmed, remember these simple tips:

Eat more vegetables and fiber.
Avoid highly processed foods.
Avoid foods with lots of salt, saturated fat, or sugar.
Drink more water and less alcohol.
Be mindful of how food is connected to your emotions.

Three Big Diet Myths We Want to Address:

1. *Eating a healthy diet is expensive.* Yes, you can spend hundreds of dollars on a week's worth of groceries. But you do not need to.

The USDA has healthy food plans available for every budget.[7] There are many resources, from individuals to organizations, that provide great tips and tricks for eating healthy on any budget.

2. *There is a "best diet" that suits everyone.* Your dietary needs, food sensitivities, digestive health, and access to food will change during your life. Knowing how to change your diet to improve your symptoms is empowering, but it can also be overwhelming. You don't have to make all these changes today, and there is no best way to do it. Take it one step at a time.

3. *A low-fat diet is best.* This myth persists despite strong evidence to the contrary. In fact, healthy fats are good for you. Low-fat diets, popularized in the 1960s, were thought to decrease heart disease and result in weight loss. Now we know more about different types of fats and the dangers of processed foods and added sugars. Low-fat diets do not prevent heart disease or lower cancer risk. Heart disease is still the number-one cause of death in high-income countries, but the number of deaths has fallen by half over the last fifty years. This decline, however, is largely due to treatment of high blood pressure and high cholesterol and a decrease in smoking rates, *not to low-fat diets.* Strong evidence indicates that the Mediterranean diet and others detailed in this chapter are healthier than a low-fat diet. So please indulge in healthy fats—they are good for you.

One important point: There isn't a best, one-size-fits-all diet for everyone, but generally a plant-based diet low in processed foods, sugar, and salt is an ideal framework to start from.

Emotions and Food

Emotions in long illness can be big: shame, pain, anger, distrust, and despair (to name a few). Food can be pleasurable and comforting. It can feel like the only way to sustain energy if you are depleted. There may be times when eating sugary or processed foods gets you through the day.

We all need comfort, especially those dealing with long illness. Sometimes a basket of fries or a slice of cake feels like the only thing that really helps. The problem is that, if consumed frequently enough, some foods are more harmful than helpful. Reflecting on how you use food as a coping mechanism can be a first step toward understanding how you cope with stress and long illness. Refer to our section on coping mechanisms (page 190) to see if there are other ways you could cope before turning to food. Another strategy is to find healthy foods that are comforting and mimic the foods that you crave most. For example:

Foods You Crave	Healthy Substitutes
Candy bar	¼ bar of dark chocolate with a handful of berries
Fries	1 cup of sweet potato fries baked with olive oil
Hamburger on a white bun	Veggie burger on a whole-wheat bun
Potato chips	1 cup of edamame beans with a pinch of sea salt

Relationships with food that are not health-promoting can be found on a spectrum with many eating disorders. Some people restrict food as a way of maintaining control. Those who overeat or undereat because of intense feelings of guilt and shame around food and weight may be simply intensifying their need for medicating with food. Food aversions and sensitivities can prompt shame and isolation.

For some people, food feels more like a tormentor than a healer, and many benefit from professional help. Addressing your underlying feelings and understanding this relationship can unlock the healing that comes from food. Connecting with a therapist who specializes in disordered eating or an experienced nutritionist is a good place to start. If you have accessibility issues or want to work on it yourself first, check out the workbook suggestions and more in our resources section.

Shifting your relationship with food is possible. In time, healthy food in a satiated body can rewire the brain. Understanding the psychological underpinnings, your relationship with food, can help.

What If You Have Trouble Accessing Food?

For many people, accessing food is a struggle. If there are times when you have difficulty getting healthy food, you are not alone. In the United States more than 10 percent of people are food-insecure—that is, they lack consistent access to adequate amounts of high-quality food. For people experiencing food insecurity, sustaining a healthy dietary eating pattern is hard without social resources and community support. We know that some of our suggestions here may be harder to follow if you are struggling. Please check out the resources section for more on food accessibility and affordable healthy food.

What Is a Healthy Dietary Eating Pattern?

A healthy dietary eating pattern is consuming foods and beverages that are high in nutrients, prevent or delay disease, and decrease symptoms of illness through adequate nutrition. There are several examples of eating this way, including the standard US-style dietary eating pattern, which shares the same core elements as more tailored eating patterns such as the popular Healthy Mediterranean-Style Dietary Pattern, the Healthy Vegetarian Dietary Pattern, and the DASH Dietary Pattern described here.

Healthy Mediterranean-Style Dietary Pattern

The Healthy Mediterranean-Style Dietary Pattern is primarily plant-based, rich in minimally processed vegetables, fruits, nuts, seeds, legumes, and unrefined grains, and high in olive oil as a primary source of fat; it includes some low-fat or fermented dairy, eggs, fish, and poultry. The diet limits, or recommends removing, red meat, processed meats, whole-fat dairy, processed foods, sugars, sweetened beverages (including juice), sodium, refined carbohydrates, and saturated fats.

The Mediterranean diet has numerous health benefits, including longer life span, lower rates of cancer mortality, and lower rates of several types of cancer. The diet helps reduce heart disease and reduces complications in people who have had heart attacks; reduces the incidence of diabetes and is helpful with diabetes management; prevents obesity and promotes weight loss and the maintenance of a healthy weight; and allows for better management of cholesterol, blood pressure, and inflammatory markers. In pregnancy, following a Mediterranean diet lowers the risk of preterm birth and fetal growth restriction. The diet is great for our brains, lowering the risks of dementia, Parkinson's disease, and Alzheimer's disease, reducing stroke risk, and delaying cognitive decline.

Healthy Vegetarian Dietary Pattern

A vegetarian way of eating doesn't include meat, but it does include animal products such as dairy (lacto) and eggs (ovo). It is different from vegan or plant-based diet variations that cut out dairy, eggs, and other animal products. Lacto-ovo-vegetarian diets are higher in micronutrients and fiber than meat-based diets and lower in calories, saturated fat, and sodium. Vitamin B_{12} and zinc are two exceptions: these micronutrients are found in high amounts in animal products but are lower in vegetarian diets.

Studies have shown that vegetarians are not deficient in calcium, iron, and protein from a vegetarian diet. In fact, eating a diet higher in plant-based proteins (instead of red or processed meats) is associated with lower mortality rates, including those related to cancer and cardiovascular disease. The overall dietary habits of vegetarians help them avoid chronic disease and reduce their long-term risk for many diseases.

If you want to increase the micronutrients that are lower in vegetarian diets (B_{12} and zinc especially) or increase your protein (if you are trying to build muscle or support fat loss), see the sections of Chapter 17 on micronutrients and on energy metabolism. Most vegetarians are able to get B_{12} from their usual diet, but vegans will need to be more intentional about eating foods high in or fortified with B_{12} and may need to take a supplement if their diet doesn't routinely include those foods.

To optimize the benefits of a vegetarian diet, you need to eat more plants. Plant-based diets have been shown to decrease inflammation and are associated with reduced incidence of some conditions, including autoimmune diseases (multiple sclerosis, rheumatoid arthritis, Graves' disease) and diabetes. Plants are full of antioxidants, which can dial down inflammation. High in fiber, plants promote a healthy microbiome. This more diverse and happier ecosystem produces more bacteria that make short-chain fatty acids, which improve your overall health by supporting your immune system, heart, and brain. Finally, plant-based diets cost less than diets that include meat, dairy, and most processed foods, which are much more expensive than their plant-based, nonprocessed counterparts.

The numerous health benefits of a vegetarian diet include the following:

Lower risk of coronary heart disease and death from heart disease
Decreased all-cause mortality, death from cancer, and death from cardiovascular disease
Decreased obesity and type 2 diabetes
Reduced risk of colorectal cancer
Lower total cholesterol, lower LDL, and higher HDL
Lower blood pressure

DASH Dietary Pattern

The Dietary Approaches to Stop Hypertension (DASH) diet was first studied to help control high blood pressure and has since been found to reduce risk for gout, heart disease, diabetes, and kidney disease. It is one of the most common dietary plans recommended by practitioners because over 50 percent of US adults have elevated blood pressure (above 120/80 mmHg). Dietary changes are one way to decrease your blood pressure; in fact, just a few weeks on the DASH diet can decrease your systolic blood pressure by around ten points. That's a big difference and reduces damage to your heart, brain, kidneys, and eyes.

DASH diet plans increase fruits, vegetables, low-fat milk, whole grains, fish, beans, nuts, and poultry, while eliminating drinks with added sugars, juice, sugary treats, and red meat. The diet focuses on reducing the level of sodium intake to less than 2,300 milligrams; it can also help some lower their cholesterol.

When you cut down on sodium, you cut out many processed and packaged foods, which also decreases added sugars and unhealthy fats. Substantial weight loss is not common on the DASH diet, but some who stick to a reduced-calorie version of it can expect some weight loss. The National Heart, Lung, and Blood Institute website offers free guidelines for picking the best DASH plan for your own needs, including menus, recipes, and food-tracking worksheets.[8] Other apps and resources are also available, and many are free.

Tips for Improving Your Anti-Inflammatory Diet

An anti-inflammatory diet increases your consumption of anti-inflammatory foods and cuts down on the pro-inflammatory foods in your diet, such as fried foods, refined carbohydrates (for example, white bread and pastries), sweetened drinks, red and processed meats, and certain fats (margarine, lard, shortening). The research is clear: inflammation from pro-inflammatory foods is associated with an increased risk of neurodegenerative disease, stroke, cancers, diabetes, heart disease, and obesity. The Mediterranean, vegetarian, and DASH diets are all anti-inflammatory diets supported by a wealth of evidence of their pro-health benefits.

Goal	Diet Changes
Increase fiber Note: If you are temporarily following an eating plan tailored to a GI issue, follow that plan.	Add high-fiber fruits and vegetables to your diet. Also increase beans, legumes, nuts, and seeds, and replace refined grains with whole grains. Aim for 25–40 grams of fiber daily, slowly increasing to avoid bowel issues.

Increase phytonutrients	Eat the rainbow to get different phytonutrients, the more colors the better. Add spices to your meals like ginger, garlic, cinnamon, turmeric, and pepper. Drink green tea and black coffee (if you use caffeine already), include soy in your diet if you can tolerate it, and choose organic when possible.
Opt for healthy fats	Eat avocados and nuts and seeds (flaxseeds, walnuts, cashews, almonds). Get omega-3 fatty acids from eating fatty fish like salmon and sardines, fortified eggs, hemp seeds, and flaxseeds. Stick to the mono-unsaturated fatty acids in oils like olive oil, canola oil, and sesame oil, and avoid hydrogenated oils, margarine, and vegetable shortening.

Specific Foods to Include in an Anti-Inflammatory Diet

Although many of the foods consumed in healthy eating patterns are anti-inflammatory, some practitioners suggest optimizing the diet by increasing particular foods. Research has shown that mushrooms, tea, dark chocolate, healthy herbs and spices, and soy have a variety of health benefits, and they are featured in some anti-inflammatory diet plans. However, we recommend that you avoid anti-inflammatory diet plans that are selling you teas or detoxes, as your body can naturally detoxify through dietary changes alone.

Mushrooms (for example, button, cremini, maitake, oyster, portobello, shiitake)	Mushrooms are a good source of selenium, copper, potassium, phosphorus, B vitamins, and, if exposed to the sun or UV light, vitamin D. They may have anti-inflammatory, antioxidant, and anti-cancer effects, and some types stimulate the immune system, protect the brain against cognitive impairment, and act as a prebiotic to support gut health.
Soy	Soy is rich in omega-3 fatty acids, phytonutrients (isoflavones), iron, zinc, B vitamins, fiber, and protein and is sometimes enriched with vitamin B_{12}, calcium, and vitamin D to support vegetarian diets. Stick mostly to whole soy foods, like edamame, tofu, yuba, and soy milk. Other soy products are okay (like veggie burgers, fake chicken, or soy protein bars), but most are highly processed and have additives and preservatives that should be avoided when possible. The evidence for exactly who should eat soy, and how much, is unclear. Some studies have shown a reduction in heart disease risk, menopause-related hot flashes, blood pressure, cholesterol, and certain types of cancer. News reports had linked soy to higher breast cancer incidence decades ago, but more recent large-scale studies in humans have shown that soy is safe and might be protective against breast cancer.

Chocolate	Chocolate is rich in flavanols, and there is strong evidence that eating high-cocoa-content (more than 70 percent) and low-sugar dark chocolate helps prevent heart disease and improve vascular health and cognitive performance. Eat no more than one ounce daily to avoid too much sugar and saturated fat.
Spices and herbs	Herbs (the leaves of the plant) and spices (the seeds of the plant, ground or whole) have shown multiple health benefits. For example: Black pepper helps with brain and joint health. Ginger can help reduce joint pain and nausea. Turmeric is helpful in many conditions, especially when paired with black pepper. Capsaicin (found in hot peppers) can slow cancer growth, heart disease, and dementia. Cinnamon helps with blood sugar, cancer, dementia, and neurodegenerative disease. Basil is antimicrobial and can help with aches and pain. Nutmeg helps to elevate mood. Anise/fennel can ease colic or gas pain. Look up your other favorite spices and herbs to learn their health benefits.
Tea	Most teas are high in polyphenols, which lower inflammation, lessen diabetes symptoms, and slow cancer growth. There are several varieties of tea. (If you are sensitive to caffeine, don't consume green or black tea past the late afternoon, when it could affect your sleep.) Herbal teas have no caffeine and are often paired with other herbs, fruits, spices, and plants with calming properties. Depending on the herbal tea you choose, it may help with cramps, spasms, stress, allergies, circulation, motion sickness, or nausea and reduce your craving for sugar. Green tea is the highest in flavonoids that boost heart health and also may decrease certain types of cancer. Matcha tea is made from green tea leaves and has the highest amount of antioxidants of all teas. People with anemia should limit their consumption of green tea, as it can reduce iron levels. Oolong tea has polyphenols and L-theanine, a protein that may reduce anxiety, increase attention, and protect against dementia. Black tea has caffeine. It can be used in baths and compresses and is used to reduce swelling, decrease pain, and decrease skin inflammation.

Should You Try Intermittent Fasting?

Intermittent fasting is a term that encompasses many techniques meant to promote mitochondrial fuel switching, or metabolic flexibility in cells.

Recall that your mitochondria can switch between different fuel types, a concept known as metabolic flexibility, which allows your body to adapt to different situations. Intermittent fasting is like stretching for your mitochondria. It pushes your mitochondria into a state of using up sugar supplies so they have to resort to breaking down fats. The breakdown of fatty acids makes ketone bodies. Ketone bodies make energy in the cell, help cells communicate, help cells reorganize and clean up, improve the performance of cells, increase the stress resistance of cells, decrease inflammation, increase antioxidant activity, and allow brain cells to grow and make new connections.

Intermittent fasting has impressive health effects:

Intermittent fasting improves the symptoms, onset, and progression of various conditions. People with asthma, rheumatoid arthritis, multiple sclerosis, Parkinson's disease, Alzheimer's disease, or cancer who intermittently fast can delay disease onset and progression and may decrease symptoms, probably because inflammation is reduced.

Intermittent fasting does more than just lose fat. People who intermittently fast lose the same amount of weight as those who simply cut calories. However, those who fast lose more belly fat and have significantly improved metabolic and inflammatory markers compared to mere calorie-cutters. Scared of losing muscle? Don't worry. So far studies have shown that you can cut fat with intermittent fasting without losing muscle mass.

Your brain works better. Intermittent fasting has been shown to reverse inflammatory disease effects on learning and memory and improve memory, cognition, and executive function in people with cognitive impairment.

There are several techniques you can use to get your body into a fasting state, including 5:2 intermittent fasting (fast two days a week and eat a regular diet five days), alternate-day fasting, and restricting daily eating time to a window (for example, 11:00 a.m.–7:00 p.m.). Generally, the last option, decreasing the time window when you eat, is a good start. The goal is to get to fasting sixteen to eighteen hours, while eating during a window of six to eight hours daily.

As you can imagine, many people are hungry and irritable when they increase their fasting time, but they become less so after a few weeks. Surprisingly, in research studies, most participants were able to stick to the fasting diet during the study, suggesting that with support intermittent fasting isn't that difficult to maintain. Check out our resources section to learn more. Loop in your practitioners to see if they have any insight, especially if you are sensitive to changes in your routine.

What About Low-Carb Diets? Or High-Protein Diets?

Many people have had a friend or family member who touts the powers of their low-carb diet. With these long-popular low-carb diets, often referred to as "keto" or "Atkins" diets, more of your calories come from fat and protein, and if your carbohydrate intake is low enough, your body might switch fuel sources to burn fat, producing ketone bodies. There are a few things to watch out for if you are going to try one of these diets.

In medical communities, ketogenic diets are used to treat a few medical conditions, like epilepsy. However, the high-fat, low-carbohydrate diet has many side effects that make it dangerous in some long illnesses. Although helpful for short-term weight loss, low-carbohydrate diets have not been shown to provide sustained weight loss. It is hard for many people to avoid their favorite foods for long periods of time. Also, those who adhere to this diet and eat more animal protein and saturated fat have higher mortality rates than those who eat other diets, including low-carb with low saturated fat. Mortality rates do not rise for people who follow low-carb plant-based diets. If your diet is high in animal protein, keep an eye on your saturated fat and try to include plant proteins.

Some people suggest keeping carbohydrates low as a way to mimic fasting, but this strategy has not been backed up by any evidence that it works.

Your mitochondria are smart and highly evolved to switch between using sugars and fats as fuels. Aside from the difficulty of maintaining a very low intake of carbohydrates, keto diets are usually high in foods with too much saturated fat, salt, red and processed meat, dairy, and processed food. For these reasons, low-carb diets are not our go-to for those with long illness.

Diets for Specific Symptoms

Elimination Diet

Some people's symptoms continue to bother them even when they are on an anti-inflammatory diet. For many different reasons, they might have become sensitive to or unable to tolerate certain foods they once were able to eat regularly. Typically, we think of "food allergies" as an immediate reaction. You eat something and immediately experience hives, swelling, or difficulty breathing. These are symptoms of true food allergies. A tremendous amount of research into food allergies in the last several decades has resulted in treatments for some of these once-fatal conditions. Allergies to specific foods, called *type 1 hypersensitivity reactions*, are best diagnosed and treated by a practitioner of allergy and immunology, usually a physician with advanced training.

However, there is more than one way to be sensitive to food. When a food makes us sick, we often use the word *allergy* when we really mean *intolerance*. An intolerance might be a reaction that happens after eating a food or a combination of foods. The reaction may depend on the amount you ate, symptoms may start days later, or they may snowball over time. When your gastrointestinal tract is inflamed, you might become more sensitive to certain foods. There are many tests for food sensitivity, but currently available tests are not always reliable. If you're interested in finding out possible triggers for your food sensitivities, the most effective way is an elimination diet.

Elimination diets cut out certain foods known to cause sensitivities, like wheat, dairy, eggs, refined sugars, corn, citrus, coffee, tea, alcohol, food additives, peanuts, and shellfish. You choose a food to eliminate from your diet to see if it is the cause of your pain, distress, or reaction. For a few days, your long illness symptoms may worsen, or you may experience fatigue, hunger, and headaches, but these symptoms usually improve. After two to three weeks, the food irritant is mostly out of your body. You then reintroduce the eliminated foods one at a time so that you know exactly what your triggers are and what to eliminate.

THE STEPS OF AN ELIMINATION DIET

Plan	Start a food journal. Write down what you eat in a week and your symptoms. Meet with your practitioner to talk about your interest in an elimination diet. Keep a list of foods you suspect of causing an issue. If there are foods that you think are triggering your symptoms, the diet is easier to follow and more likely to work.
Prepare	Get rid of foods you will be eliminating from your home and other places you eat. Plan out your meals and grocery lists. Plan on eating your own food for the next two to four weeks, avoid travel, and schedule social and life events accordingly. Tell your friends and family about your plan and ask for support. Make sure you are mentally, financially, and physically prepared to undertake this diet.
Eliminate	The first few days you might experience withdrawal from sugars, caffeine, and other substances your body is used to. This will pass. Try to eat unprocessed foods to avoid hidden ingredients. After a week, you might notice a reduction of your symptoms. Keep tabs on your symptoms during the elimination phase. Most symptoms should be gone after two weeks, but it might take up to four weeks. If there is no change, consider cutting out different foods.
Challenge	After five days without symptoms, add back foods one at a time. Continue your food and symptom journal. Every three days add back more of the food you eliminated. For example, on day one eat one blueberry, on day two eat six blueberries, and on day three eat twenty blueberries. If you have a reaction, put that food on your avoid list. If you aren't sure, cut it out once again and then make another attempt to add it either after you are done reintroducing all the other foods or in five days.
New diet	You now should have a list of foods that trigger symptoms and what those symptoms are. You can continue with your previous diet, being careful to avoid the foods that cause issues. Continue to keep a symptom journal, and if they return, track the foods you eat again and repeat this process. Always involve a practitioner in your findings so they can help guide you.

If you find yourself cutting out many foods, fearing foods, or not enjoying eating, you need to involve your practitioner to get you on track. Elimination diets can ignite disordered eating patterns, so be honest with yourself and your practitioners if you are having negative thoughts or feelings about food and eating. *People who use alcohol regularly or heavily, have a history of eating disorders or a current eating disorder, are underweight or malnourished, experience OCD, or are at risk for severe allergic reaction (severe atopic dermatitis and asthma) should consider eliminating substances from their diet only with the advice and monitoring of their health care team to avoid possibly life-threatening situations.*

Elimination diets are hard, both to carry out and to interpret. You might not get clear answers, and that is okay. An elimination diet is just another tool for learning more about your symptoms and may not be right for everyone. Make sure you are ready and have practitioners who are on board for any hiccups or hitches along this path.

Autoimmune Protocol (AIP) Diet

This diet, which combines principles of paleo and elimination diets, is popular among people with autoimmune disease who want to get better control of their symptoms. Foods that have been associated with increased gut permeability ("leaky gut"), including legumes, grains, nuts, seeds, oils, nightshades, eggs, dairy, refined and processed foods, sugars, alcohol, and coffee, are eliminated. Some medications are also discontinued. The AIP diet is very restrictive, and many people find it hard to follow for long periods of time.

The diet consists mainly of meat, fermented foods, bone broth, fruit, and vegetables. It also includes a large lifestyle component of stress reduction, sleep improvement, and exercise, all of which contributes to improved quality of life. After an elimination diet of one to three months, foods are reintroduced one at a time. If a food results in symptoms, it is removed from the diet moving forward.

An issue with cutting out foods permanently is that your food tolerance can change over time. We suggest that, unless you have a true food allergy diagnosed by an allergist, you try reintroducing foods more than once, so that you don't limit your diet forever. With many of these diets, some people are fearful about adding foods back once symptoms have improved. With the support of multiple practitioners, you should be able to find the most well rounded and least restricted diet for yourself. Most sensitivities to foods suggest that the body can't handle certain amounts of substances at particular moments in time. But bodies constantly change. Although it is scary, be open to reintroducing foods you have cut out, not only because it is important to have a healthy relationship with food, but also because restricted diets can be harmful, cause nutrient deficiencies, and lead to social isolation.

Aside from being difficult to follow and restrictive, the AIP diet is not well supported by research because few studies have been conducted. What results we have show slight improvement in symptoms but no change in inflammatory or disease-related markers. By contrast, the multiple health benefits of a Mediterranean, vegetarian, or DASH diet are supported by strong data, which is why they are recommended as long-term diets. The autoimmune protocol might appeal to those who are interested in doing an autoimmune disease or ketogenic-themed elimination diet. There is no evidence, however, that it is better than the standard elimination diet.

Free Radicals and Diet

Free radicals are normal products of metabolism, made in the mitochondria. You can also be exposed to them in the environment of the foods you eat (fats, sugars, processed food), alcohol, pollution, sun exposure (radiation), smoking, or toxins (such as pesticides). Free radical molecules exist for less than a second but can cause significant changes to nearby fat, protein, and DNA. In the bloodstream, they fight off pathogens (like bacteria) and help with many other tasks in the body. But they also can cause trouble. Damage from free radicals, known as oxidative stress, causes many health issues like arthritis, vision loss, heart disease, cancers, and acceleration of aging.

Your mitochondria have a cleanup crew that helps protect them from the unwieldy free radicals: antioxidants. Your body makes a small amount of antioxidants by itself, but you need to eat foods high in antioxidants to get enough. An anti-inflammatory diet high in antioxidants like vitamins A, C, and E, lutein, lycopene, and other nutrients is critical to keeping your mitochondria healthy.

We strongly recommend that you get your antioxidants from food. The supplements out there just don't compare to what food can offer. For example, there are eight types of vitamin E in food, but only one has been researched and is widely available as a supplement. Food also has other benefits, like fiber and other nutrients. Plus, eating makes you feel good!

Some antioxidant supplements can be toxic at high levels. According to large studies, most antioxidant supplements do not reduce your risk of developing disease, and some high-dose antioxidants can increase your risk of cancer and stroke. Make sure you check in with your medical team before taking unnecessary supplements that you can get from a handful of nuts and berries.

Eating Your Antioxidants

Increasing the antioxidants you eat supports your mitochondrial functioning. As you read through this list of antioxidants, take note of what you are already including in your diet. What are some of your favorite foods that include these antioxidants? Do you see any foods here that you want to try to add to your diet? Try to eat foods from each group to get a variety of antioxidants. Some foods have multiple antioxidants. Keep in mind that this is a list of just some of the foods you can eat to increase your antioxidant intake.

Flavonoids	Black tea, green tea, citrus fruits, red wine, onions, berries, apples, red cabbage
Isoflavonoids	Soybeans, tofu, lentils, peas, milk
Polyphenols	Pomegranates, olive oil, flax, grapes, oregano, dark chocolate, pecans, legumes, teas
Vitamin C	Citrus fruits, kiwi, mangoes, broccoli, spinach, berries, peppers
Vitamin E	Avocados, nuts, seeds, tomatoes, mangoes
Allium sulfur	Leeks, onions, garlic, chives

Anthocyanins	Purple foods like eggplant, grapes, berries, red cabbage
Beta-carotene	Pumpkin, mangoes, apricots, carrots, spinach, parsley
Catechins	Red wine, tea, blueberries, kiwi, cacao
Copper	Seafood, lean meat, milk, nuts
Cryptoxanthins	Orange foods like pumpkin, mangoes, oranges, pineapple, peaches, corn
Indoles	Cruciferous vegetables like broccoli, cabbage, cauliflower, turnips, Brussels sprouts
Lignans	Flaxseed, sesame seeds, bran, whole grains, vegetables
Lutein	Green-yellow foods like corn, spinach, kale, collards, pumpkin, eggs, carrots
Lycopene	Red-pink foods like tomatoes, pink grapefruit, watermelon, papaya
Manganese	Seafood, lean meat, milk, nuts
Selenium	Seafood, lean meat, whole grains
Vitamin A	Liver, sweet potatoes, carrots, milk, egg yolks, broccoli, apricots
Zinc	Seafood, lean meat, milk, nuts

EXERCISE

INCREASE YOUR ANTIOXIDANTS

Some of your favorite foods are full of antioxidants. Here are some ideas to increase your intake of antioxidants, one bite at a time. Which one will you try this week? What antioxidant-rich foods can you add to recipes you already make regularly to increase the antioxidants you eat in a week?

TIPS

Shifting Your Eating Patterns

No matter what eating pattern you decide to follow, here are some suggestions to make the transition easier:

- **Make gradual changes.** When increasing your fruits, vegetables, and legumes, you may experience an increase in gas and bloating. If this happens, consider making these changes more gradually. These symptoms are unlikely to persist, and your body just needs time to adjust.

- **Don't let yourself get too hungry.** If you are hungry enough, your brain may worry that you are going to starve. Starvation cues the brain to shut down control mechanisms for regulating how much you eat, and as a result you may eat large volumes of food without sensing fullness. Try to use healthy snack foods (listed here) to help your system sense when you are full.

- **Plan ahead.** If you are going out to eat or to a friend's house, check ahead to see what food will be available and make a plan for what you are going to eat. Some people are stigmatized for having dietary limitations, but most of us know someone trying to make dietary changes and will support them and encourage their journey to improve their health.

- **Hang out with people who support you.** It takes a few months for your new eating patterns to stick. Get your friends on board with your change. If they are not accommodating, hang out with them in situations where no food is involved.

    Be gentle with yourself. No one is perfect. This isn't about eating everything exactly right. Small shifts can make for big changes in health. Aim for progress, not perfection.

TIPS

Keeping on Top of Your Diet When You Have a Chronic Illness
Stock up on:

- **Frozen vegetables and fruit:** They are fresh and nutritious (as they are frozen right after being picked). Keep your freezer stocked with your favorites.

- **Healthy snacks:** Some easy favorites include hummus with carrot and celery sticks; avocado and red pepper slices; apple or banana with almond butter; cottage cheese with pineapple; a handful of nuts, seeds, and berries; dark chocolate (more than 70 percent cocoa); edamame beans; and smoothies.

- **Other great high-quality foods:** Nuts and seeds, unflavored, raw, and unsalted if possible; nut butters (aim for those made only with nuts); canned vegetables and legumes such as beans, lentils, tomatoes, and corn (with BPA-free lining if possible); brown, whole-grain, or black rice (available in rapid-cook forms); oats; and canned fish (tuna, sardines, salmon).

What else do you like to keep stocked in your pantry?

TIPS

Keep a Handle on Your Symptoms, Optimize Absorptions, and Curb Your Cravings

- If you are able, eat four to six small meals during the day, every four to five hours, instead of large meals. (This will look different for each person.)
- At each eating time eat at least 10 to 20 grams of protein (unless you've been prescribed a low-protein diet). Aim for at least 0.8 times your weight in kilograms (1 kilogram = 2.2 pounds). For example, if you weigh 70 kilograms (154 pounds), you should get 70 kilograms x 0.8 grams per kilogram = 56 grams of protein a day. We recommend more protein for people who have a long illness and people who are physically active.
- If nausea is an issue, sip cool beverages, use anti-nausea medications before eating, and use ginger to settle your stomach. Try eating foods with less odor, typically cold or room-temperature foods. Drinking peppermint tea with your meals and timing medications that cause or help nausea around meals can be helpful in managing your nausea.
- Shop for and plan meals when you are full and feeling well to support well-thought-out choices. When you are feeling badly, set yourself up to win by identifying a meal from food delivery or an easy meal to make at home that is simple and healthy.
- When you're having good days, cook in bulk. Divide the prepared food into servings in containers and freeze for easy meals later.

- If your friends or loved ones want to help, let them. Keep your pantry stocked and a list of your favorites on your fridge in case someone needs to shop for you. They can help keep you accountable to your anti-inflammatory diet.
- Depending on your illness and income, you might be eligible for home support funded by the government. See the resources section for more information and ask your primary care practitioner if you might qualify. Communities often have a food bank or food delivery services for which people with chronic illness can qualify. This can be helpful if you are recovering from a hospitalization or flare-up.
- Indulge yourself from time to time. It's okay to eat your favorite treat occasionally.
- Drink lots of water during the day, but not immediately before or during a meal. Drink what you need to lubricate your food, but not much more. We recommend drinking two glasses of water about an hour before you are planning to eat to ensure that you are hydrated while you eat.

Questions for Your Medical Team

To discover how your health care practitioners can reinforce the positive changes you are making in your life, ask them the following questions:

Are there any foods, macronutrients, or nutrients I need to limit? (For example, some people need low or high protein, and some should avoid lactose.)

Are there any changes you would make to my diet that you recommend to other people with my illness?

Are there certain dietary plans that you would not want me to do because of my medical condition?

What kinds of support or resources can you provide to help me stay on my diet? Can you connect me with classes to learn more about cooking or diet, access to affordable, healthy foods, or food delivery when I am sick?

When I am feeling sick, are there certain things you think I should eat more or less of?

I'm trying to lose a significant amount of fat. Is a referral to a weight management practitioner appropriate for me?

(*If your practitioner is unable to answer these questions*) Who else can I speak with to learn more?

CHAPTER 19

Explore Movement for Body and Soul

The message that I would give to people struggling with exercise is that you have a really big project. You need to get attuned to your body signals so that you can recognize when you need to stop and you can figure out what kind of activity you can do that will keep you within your limits. But the most important thing is to not crash. Finding ways to engage your muscles and keep moving, even if you are bedbound, is really valuable and makes a big difference to your body.

You might read this opening quotation and think, "Well, that's all fine— but I am in pain and have mobility issues. Exercise? It's hard enough to just do daily life." And we hear you. We know from discussions with many people with long illness that it can be frustrating to hear, "Just move. You'll feel better!" The good news is that movement can happen anytime and anywhere—and pretty much all movement counts as exercise, even deep breathing or stretching in bed.

What You Will Learn in This Chapter:

- The different ways a body can move and reap the benefits
- The compelling reasons to use exercise as medicine
- Ways to engage with movement that feels tailored to your body
- Tips to cultivate motivation and get moving!

There are two major types of exercise: aerobic and anaerobic training. In aerobic training, you use muscles more than you usually would, increasing your heart rate and use of oxygen. Aerobic exercise includes running, cycling, and dancing, but also sweeping, walking to work, and running errands. Anaerobic exercise is aimed at increasing your strength, balance, and coordination by using your body weight or adding additional weight. Doing push-ups or squats or lifting weights are traditional examples, but other ways of moving around your house in your day-to-day life, such as picking up a child or a pet, can count as resistance exercise. Other types of exercise are aimed at specific skills such as coordination, balance, flexibility, agility, speed, and power. You might not have thought of many movements you do regularly as exercise, but it all adds up.

For some people, the thought of being able to increase how much they exercise makes them laugh out loud. With a long illness, there will be times when you wish you could exercise but you can't. There will be times when you hit all your exercise goals and still feel bad. A movement that is easy today might be impossible tomorrow. In these moments, remember: exercise is worth it. You might not feel it or appreciate it immediately, and sometimes you might be sore or more tired from exercise, but the evidence of the positive long-term effects from movement are rock-solid.

We get it: moving enough every day is not easy for most people. But recent research has some good news: even just a few more minutes of moving a day can give you some of these health benefits. Each year new studies show more health benefits of exercise. From preventing disease to slowing disease progression, decreasing symptom burden, and improving how we feel about ourselves and our lives, the benefits are significant. You don't have to make it to the ideal amount of movement. You just need to take baby steps to move more.

EVIDENCE-BASED BENEFITS OF EXERCISE FOR ADULTS

Lowers Risk of	Reduces	Improves
Most types of deaths	Symptoms of depression	Quality of life
Hypertension, type 2 diabetes, and adverse blood lipid profile	Symptoms of anxiety	Thinking and memory
Dementia, Alzheimer's disease, and neurodegenerative disorders	Disease progression of diabetes and hypertension	Sleep quality

Depression and anxiety	Weight gain, both initially and after weight loss, and osteoarthritis pain	Bone health
Cardiovascular disease, including heart disease and stroke, and mortality from these diseases	Inflammation, overall and long-term	Self-esteem
Cancer of the bladder, breast, colon, endometrium, esophagus, kidney, lung, and stomach	Fatigue	Cognition and memory
Falls in older adults and fall-related injuries in older adults	Effects of stress	Physical function
Postpartum depression, excessive weight gain, and gestational diabetes in pregnancy		Energy

How Much Should You Be Exercising?

For eighteen- to sixty-four-year-olds of all abilities and conditions, whether they have end-stage breast cancer or compete as Olympic athletes, whether they're bedbound or always on the move, the recommendations for how much exercise they need are the same. Moving from "no activity" to "some levels" provides you with health benefits, and those benefits keep increasing as you get to your goal. You might need to adjust the recommendations based on your own exercise capacity, health risks, or limitations, but with time you will get stronger and it will get easier.

Type of Exercise	Frequency	Increased Benefits Up to...
Aerobic: Moderate intensity[a]	150 minutes at least once a week	300 minutes
Aerobic: Vigorous intensity[b]	75 minutes at least once a week	150 minutes
Anaerobic: Muscle strengthening[c]	2 days, 15–30 minutes each day	Any additional days

[a] *Increased heart rate—can talk but can't sing.*
[b] *Increased heart rate—can't talk without stopping to catch breath.*
[c] *Any activity that works all the major muscle groups harder than normal.*

Just remember that what 150 minutes of moderate exercise looks like for you is not going to look the same for your friends—or even your twin—and that is okay! Like everything else recommended in this book, moderation and small steps are key.

If you have a long illness, doing long, high-intensity exercise can be harder on your body than it is for others. Ideally, you should try to space out your exercise over the week. If you do all your exercise on the weekend, that is okay, but people who exercise a little bit daily are more likely to keep up that habit in the long run. Try to incorporate active travel into your day, like walking or cycling to get around. You can also spread your household chores throughout the week and exercise during passive activities like watching TV or reading.

Talk to your health care team about the physical activities you should be doing for your condition and situation. Recommendations from your team should change and adapt over time based on your abilities and situation. You can talk to your team now about how to be prepared to exercise in certain situations, like being bedbound or in the hospital, or when you are trying to increase your fitness goals. It is important to keep moving even when you are feeling sick or you're in the hospital. Every day that you are inactive you lose muscle and functional ability.

That is why a nurse will get you up out of bed and put you in a chair, or a physical therapist will walk with you. Studies have shown that increased physical activity after discharge improves sleep and recovery time, decreases readmission rates, and increases survival.

EXERCISE

IT ALL ADDS UP

Every movement we make contributes to our health. Review this list of different ways to incorporate exercise into your day. In your journal, write down in one column the activities you do regularly; in another column write down the activities you might want to try or do more of.

Walking	Vacuuming	Rowing	Gardening	Doing dishes
Cooking	Cycling	Moving furniture	Water aerobics	Hunting
Cardio classes	Yoga	Swimming	Scrubbing	Pilates
Hiking	Carrying boxes	Tai chi	Tennis	Baling hay
Playing with kids	Dancing	Mopping	Lifting weights	Doing laundry
Stretching	Boxing	Golfing	Carrying bags	Shopping
Martial arts	Lawn care	Climbing stairs	Surfing	Shoveling
Kayaking	Fishing	Skiing	Jogging/running	Hula hoop
Frisbee	Table tennis	Sweeping	Soccer	Horseback riding
Wall sits	Dog walking	Balancing	Sexual activity	Basketball

Journaling

THE JOY OF EXERCISE

Think of activities or movements that make you laugh or give you joy. For some it is playing a game of basketball with their friends. For others it is going on a long walk in the woods, or cleaning their bathroom. Use the list here to brainstorm. Think of the last exercise you did that brought you joy.

> Who did you do that activity with? Where were you? What time of day was it?
>
> Write down thoughts and images that bring you back to that experience.
>
> How did you feel after you completed that activity?
>
> How did your body feel physically? Were you sweaty, hot, cold, tired, full of energy?
>
> How did you feel mentally? Strong, capable, satisfied?
>
> What do you think motivates you to do activities that bring you joy?

Why Do You Need to Do Strength or Resistance Training?

We lose roughly 5 percent of our muscle mass each decade once we reach our thirties, and it only gets worse with lack of activity. Maintaining muscle is critical for your health. Strength training alone lowers your risk of heart attack, stroke, diabetes, cancer, and premature death, and ultimately it supports the health of your gut, bones, pancreas, blood vessels, immune system, adrenal glands, and liver and helps break down fat. Strength training is the only exercise that protects you from bone loss, lessening your risk of osteoporosis and fractures as you age. Like aerobic exercise, strength training has benefits for your brain, including improvement in memory, attention, and reaction time. Keeping your muscles strong helps prevent falls and makes problems with moving less severe.

A few years after my diagnosis that explained my arthritis, I had a bad accident where I broke over ten bones. I had a really great physical therapist. She had had an accident when she was young and had a long physical recovery herself. She was very blunt with me. She told me, "You have to be strong. If your muscles are strong, it will mean there is less stress on your joints. You need to pay attention to your muscles now." It made a huge difference in my recovery, and I believe because I was stronger, my arthritis didn't flare up as much as it would have.

When you are feeling too weak to do resistance exercises, or when you have an injury, even just imagining exercising can help prevent loss of muscle mass and ability. The act of imagining you are doing strength exercises strengthens the connections in your brain that help move your muscles. The parts of your brain that are used to do a movement also are activated when you think about doing that movement.

EXERCISE

BRAIN MOVEMENT

Imagine something you enjoy or used to enjoy doing. Maybe it was swimming in the ocean, throwing a ball around with your friends, climbing a tree, walking through your favorite neighborhood, or dancing.

Focus on that activity. Imagine yourself getting dressed, putting on your shoes, planning your route, calling your friend to join you, grabbing your keys, walking out the door. While imagining getting ready, set your goal for your imaginary movement. What will you do? Who will you do it with? What time of day is it? What is the weather like?

Start the activity. What are the smells? Tastes? Sights? Sounds? What does the air around you feel like? You feel stronger and more confident with each step. Your muscles and bones are moving quickly and nimbly, with the skill of a champion athlete and the adaptability of a child.

If doubts come into your mind, repeat a mantra that resonates with you. Pick one or make up your own: "I've got this!" "I am strong." "I believe in myself." "I am awesome."

Continue the activity in your imagination. With each movement, focus on your breathing and heart rate. Is your heart rate speeding up when you speed up? Is your breathing getting faster when you go faster? Are your muscles twitching or do they feel like they are moving?

As you finish the activity, begin to cool down. Imagine yourself stretching or relaxing after you exercise. Try adding on a progressive muscle relaxation exercise (page 178) to check in on your body.

Next time try a different activity or change up your imaginary partners or location. You might notice that the next time you actually do the activity, or a similar activity, it is easier, or you are better at it. That is because the same parts of your brain are being used and so it might actually be easier for your brain! Pretty cool, huh?

Is It Medically Safe to Exercise?

If you do dishes, walk to the bathroom, or ride a bike, then you already are exercising. We call these NEAT (Non-Exercise Activity Thermogenesis) activities. NEAT activities aren't thought of formally as exercise, but they are. If you can do these activities without shortness of breath or chest pain, then it is okay for you to continue doing them as well as other moderate-intensity exercise. Most people do not need to see a health care practitioner to increase their level of exercise, but if you have a long illness you should inform your medical team of your plans for exercise.

Your Practitioners Told You to Rest When You're Feeling Sick and Not to Exercise or Push Yourself. Is This True?

There are certain times with some conditions when you should not exercise, or you should do so only under the direct instruction and supervision of licensed professionals. Some of these situations are temporary and have usually resulted in a trip to the hospital, such as heart attacks, blood clots, collapsed lungs, or other temporary inflammation or infection of the lungs and heart. In these emergencies, or if you have an uncontrolled flare or infection, you should not be exercising. Similarly, if you have severe chronic disease of the heart and lungs, including severe pulmonary hypertension, severe narrowing of the aorta, decompensated heart failure, or a similar disease, you should not exercise until your team believes it is safe to do so.

You might think it is better to rest when you are sick or hurt. For most conditions, this is an outdated idea. Evidence has shown not only that this idea is not true, but that not moving can worsen your condition and overall health. Some practitioners might see your condition as a limitation and make recommendations based on an ableist[9] view of your condition. It is okay to educate your practitioners, especially if they haven't worked too often with people who have your type of condition. If only one practitioner tells you not to exercise, ask other members of your health care team what they think. Unless you are actively infected, or your heart and lungs are severely impaired, movement is more likely to be helpful than harmful. Movement is even helpful at the end of life and is recommended for patients receiving palliative care and in hospice, as it improves quality of life and eases symptoms.

Exercise is the most complicated because the mitochondria in my muscles don't work well. It hurts when I exercise because my lactate gets high very fast. My legs hurt, I feel dizzy. But I know that exercising is the only way to make my

good mitochondria stronger so that they can beat out the weak, sick mitochon-
dria. I like to use my spin bike, so I don't stress out my joints, and do some
strengthening exercises with my [Nintendo] Wii.

If you have post-exertional malaise or fatigue, one of the main symptoms in myalgic encephalomyelitis/chronic fatigue syndrome (ME/CFS), see Chapter 5 for a more in-depth discussion.

Things to Consider When You Are Exercising

You already have enough to deal with, long illness or not. Here are some suggestions to set yourself up for success and avoid downtime from injury or flare.

> **Protect yourself.** When appropriate, wear a helmet and protective clothing; be visible to other people; tell people your plans if you are exercising alone; wear gloves to protect your hands against temperature or injury; pick activities that are going to be most appropriate to your abilities; use appropriate ability-enhancing gear, including braces, tape, and sun-protective clothing; and consider using a heart rate monitor to ensure that your workout is as safe as possible.
>
> **Start low and go slow.** Engage in activities appropriate for your level of experience and ability. Slowly increase your intensity and duration. Monitor how your body responds and scale back or increase exercise according to how you feel.
>
> **Stay hydrated.** Make sure to drink eight to sixteen ounces of water in the hour or two before exercising. Also drink while exercising, and again afterward. Bring water with you and a snack if appropriate.
>
> **Be aware of your environment.** Heat can be difficult for some people with long illness. Exercise is improved for everyone, however, if it's done in well-ventilated areas during cooler times of the day, a fan is used to keep cool, and clothing appropriate for the weather is worn.

Stop if you feel something is off. Check in with yourself regularly. If you feel sick or strange, pause and reassess. Let your medical team know if you are experiencing any symptoms while exercising.

When Should You Talk to Your Practitioners About Physical Activity?

Every visit with every practitioner should touch on how you are getting around and how your exercise routine is going. If they don't bring it up, you should. Keep your health care team up to date on your goals and how you are doing. Goals don't have to be big. It is helpful to set small, realistic goals that you can meet. Ask your health care team for an exercise prescription and information about how you can be more physically active.

Be sure to tell your health care team if you are having any difficulties tolerating exercise (like breathlessness, fatigue, or pain). With certain conditions, specific modifications can be made to help set you up for success. No matter what your underlying condition, tracking your symptoms and exercise in a journal can enable you to notice patterns that may lead you to make modifications or to bring them up with your health care team.

What Is an Exercise Prescription?

Primary care practitioners and anyone who specializes in exercise should be able to give you an exercise prescription. For each type of exercise, they should set a FITT (frequency, intensity, time, and type of exercise) goal. FITT goals should meet you at your ability level and are likely to include— or to build up to include—exercises that address aerobics, muscles, flexibility, composition, and balance. Practitioners will talk with you about your motivations, discuss any potential barriers, and review the prescription. After a set amount of time, or if the exercises become too easy, you should check back with your practitioner to advance your prescription to a stronger dose. If you find some exercises too difficult, let your practitioner know so they can modify the recommendations.

Example Prescription for a Beginner

Frequency: Three times a week

Intensity: Moderate (can talk but not sing)

Time: Fifteen to thirty minutes

Type: Brisk walk or stationary bicycle (adapt for ability)

It's really hard to exercise when you feel tired and you're in pain. I feel like my body is prone to injury. I feel like I have the body of a seventy-five-year-old (I'm in my thirties). Exercise can be really helpful for me for my mood, if nothing else. But there is such a thing as overdoing it in my body, and if I overdo it, I feel way worse. So I have to be very gentle with how I exercise. I do try to go on walks, or hikes, gentle hikes. Again, nothing longer than like maybe an hour, nothing terribly steep or challenging, but just a nice, pleasant walk on the beach or through nature, you know. [It's] really helpful to my mood, helpful for getting endorphins going.

How Do You Exercise the Right Amount for You?

When exercise doesn't make you feel good, it's hard to do it. Pacing is a self-tailored way to modify your mental and physical activity levels according to what is going on in your body. It allows you to modify how you do an activity so you can complete it, which will increase strength, tolerance, and functional ability. With pacing, you are developing an exercise plan that enables you to hit your sweet spot so that you rest at the right time and don't feel bad after completing your activity.

Pacing sounds simple, but it is infinitely involved. Most people find it hard to always get it right. The signals that tell us we need to stop are really subtle, and the desire to get things done is often really strong. And the world doesn't accommodate the need to stop on a dime. There is a certain amount of grace to this that has to be mastered as well as possible. It is not easy.

Here is an example of what cleaning the kitchen might look like before incorporating pacing:

Pushed through fifteen minutes of cleaning up.
Felt exhausted and had back pain for an hour. Needed to stay in bed.

With pacing, cleaning the kitchen might look more like this:

Washed dishes for five minutes.
Rested for thirty minutes.
Wiped counters and put away dishes for five minutes.
Rested for thirty minutes.
Swept floor for five minutes.
Kitchen cleaned, exercised for fifteen minutes total, feel great, no flare
    or pain.

Often when you are having a good day and you're hanging out with friends or doing something you like, you might push yourself too far. Be mindful of times when you push yourself. One person with long illness learned over time not to go too hard when doing something with friends.

It took a while for me to be okay with being the slowpoke, but now I can go outside and enjoy hikes with my friends. Now if I notice that someone else is going slow, I will take a break and set an example of pacing for them. I also really pay attention to how much water I am drinking and make sure I drink water and have some snacks with me. Now I can hike for longer and am not overly tired after a long day on the trails.

Motivation

So now it's clear that movement is good for you, it can be very helpful with long illness, it doesn't have to be rigorous to be beneficial, and you need to incorporate it into your life. But how do you get yourself to actually move? Here are some tips and tricks:

Anticipate obstacles and plan ahead. If you have a plan for when you encounter a barrier, you are more likely to complete your task. For example, plan what to do if you experience a flare and need to rest before resuming movement again.

Train your brain to associate exercise with a reward. Although exercising can make you feel good, if you plan on a treat at the end of the exercise, not only are you motivated, but your brain gets more excited and the connection between the activity and pleasure is strengthened.

Put your money where your muscle is. You may be motivated by signing a commitment pledge or setting up a monetary penalty. Research has shown that using these tools can help you stick to your goals better than people who do not use them.

Spread the word. Telling people your goals or writing them down makes you more likely to complete them. Putting a sticky note on your bathroom mirror or having a friend checking in by text is a proven way to help yourself follow through on your goals.

Find your people. Whatever you enjoy, there are others out there who want to share it with you. Maybe your community has to be online owing to circumstances beyond your control, but building any type of community around movement brings major rewards for your health. Just like pairing an exercise with a reward, exercising with others adds the benefits of bonding, encouragement from others, a confidence boost, and often a bit of levity to the day. Your community can be as simple as going on a walk with your neighbor or texting a picture of yourself on a hike to a friend.

How Do You Build New Physical Activity Habits?

Keep it simple! All movement is exercise. Point and flex your toes while you are lying down or sitting. Do an extra lap around the sofa, grocery store, yard, or block.

Keep an exercise journal. Log your exercise in your symptom or food journal. This will help you learn what you can tolerate and what kind of movement decreases symptoms. You might notice that after exercising, for example, you sleep better.

Talk to your health care team. They can help you brainstorm ideas for any mobility and exercise adaptations you might need to make based on your condition, medications, or situation. Ask for referrals to exercise specialists like physical or occupational therapists, exercise trainers, or rehabilitation programs (such as cardiac, vestibular, pulmonary, or stroke rehabilitation programs), either online or in person.

Sign up for groups or classes. Committing to a movement group or exercise class helps you build a movement community and gives you routine access to a teacher who is motivated to support you in reaching your goals. It is a great way to meet other people who are on similar journeys, learn from movement teachers, avoid inactivity, and increase your motivation by being in a positive environment at least once a week. Look for walking groups in your neighborhood, online exercise classes, or local classes that you are interested in. Members of many chronic illness support groups form physical activity groups or even sports leagues. Use your illness communities to learn tips and tricks about how to exercise more easily.

Have a movement buddy. Even if you live in different places, having someone to check in with about your exercise is helpful for staying on track. Better yet, have a movement buddy nearby and commit to a goal together. Even if it is as small a commitment as going on a short walk once a week, getting yourself moving and in a supportive environment is key to motivating yourself to exercise more.

Use technology! Smartphone apps, wearable technology like smart watches and pedometers, and insurance or health system text or call programs are all aimed at giving you feedback about your activity. Most of these technologies can provide reminders and reinforcement for doing exercise.

Get going. Every hour, move around for a minute. Get your blood flowing and your heart rate up.

EXERCISE

GET MOVING

Try one of these today to get yourself moving and using different muscles or more muscles.

> *Play music and dance around in your chair, lying in bed, on the floor, around your kitchen, or outside. Our brains love music and our bodies get pleasure from dancing. When we dance to music, we feel a sense of control and power because our brains understand the patterns of music and love knowing what is coming next.*

> *Sit on the floor. It requires more muscles to sit down on the floor and get up than it does to sit in a chair. Your balance and coordination are both challenged.*

> *Clean up that pile of stuff that has been sitting around. This usually sends you all over your house and to the garbage to organize the mystery pile.*

> *Play charades or a similar game that keeps you moving. Laughter uses muscles.*

> *Walk to the store or a restaurant instead of driving. You might start a new habit and explore your neighborhood at the same time.*

What other creative ways can you think of to increase your movement?

CHAPTER 20

How Traditional Medicine Can Help Long Illness

What You Will Learn in This Chapter:

- An overview of the usefulness of traditional medicine in long illness
- An exploration of acupuncture, East Asian medicine, and Ayurvedic medicine
- Tools and concepts from traditional medicine that you can apply now
- Ways to get connected with a traditional medicine practitioner if these concepts resonate and you are looking for a different approach to care

People living with long illness can have problems throughout the body, and many are aware that it is all connected. Unfortunately, conventional biomedicine rarely appreciates these visible and invisible layers of interconnectivity. Despite seeing multiple medical specialists, you may not feel any closer to understanding *why* you feel the way you do. Adding a traditional medicine practitioner to your medical team can cultivate a new awareness and enhance healing.

Before the development of modern medicine, communities cultivated and passed on knowledge, skills, and practices based on their personal experiences with illness. We now refer to these practices as "traditional" medicine. In some countries, most primary health care is provided by following these traditions. Traditional practices have been shared across cultures, and some have been adopted by other groups or cultures, often becoming modified along the way. Over time biomedical science has tested some of these practices to find out if they can help with illness. Some studies have shown that many traditional practices are not only safe but can benefit people's health by both preventing and treating disease. Other practices have been shown to have no benefit while causing no harm, while some have been proven to be harmful.

In this chapter, we briefly explore some of the traditional practices in common use today. A mountain of detailed literature describes each of these practices, but here we simply explain the evidence behind their use and describe the symptoms they might be helpful for.

Acupuncture

> *I know I am always going to have pain because of my illness. I saw different doctors, tried lots of different medications and exercises. Then my PCP asked if I would try acupuncture. I was very skeptical because of the cost and I don't like needles. [But] I decided for six months I would try it, and it was amazing. It helped with my pain, but even more it has helped with my anxiety. It also helped me feel less nauseous.*

Acupuncture is a two-thousand-year-old technique for preventing or treating various conditions by using fine needles inserted at specific points of the body or pressure applied at those points. The locations of these points are based on traditional Chinese medicine (TCM) points that connect energy (qi) channels, called meridians. (You'll read more about TCM in just a bit.) Although once controversial in biomedical medicine, acupuncture is now widely used throughout the world. Multiple large studies have made it clear that acupuncture is safe.

Some might question whether having needles inserted in your body could be relaxing, but we encourage you to have an open mind. The needle used is very thin, and discomfort, if any, is minimal and momentary. For those of you who have a phobia of needles, *acupressure* may be a helpful alternative. With acupressure, pressure from a fingertip is used instead of a needle to target the same points on your body. A practitioner can even teach you self-acupressure to help with various symptoms.

We don't know exactly why acupuncture makes you feel better; it is difficult to draw conclusions from studies on acupuncture to date, for multiple reasons. However, the strongest evidence for its effectiveness is in people who experience chronic pain, including neck and low back pain and arthritis. Research also supports the use of acupuncture in the treatment of migraines, hot flashes, cancer-related pain, nausea from chemotherapy, surgery, pregnancy, seasonal allergies, and chronic obstructive pulmonary disease (COPD). People gain relief or improvement from acupuncture for many other conditions as well. Acupuncture is a good tool to use regularly or to put in your toolbox to use when your symptoms are overwhelming.

Acupuncture can be practiced by a licensed doctor of Asian medicine, chiropractic medicine, or dentistry who also has completed training in acupuncture.[10] The different styles of acupuncture include TCM, Japanese, Korean, auricular,[11] five elements, and medical acupuncture. We recommend having consultations with several acupuncturists before selecting one, to make sure you will work well together.

Health insurance is more frequently covering visits for acupuncture as its popularity increases. Insurance sometimes covers acupuncture for pain or nausea. Contact your health care plan to learn more about your options. There are ways to save on this sometimes costly treatment, such as using a health savings account or flex spending account, going to an acupuncturist who charges a sliding scale fee for service, asking about reduced rates or free service, or going to community acupuncture (one practitioner treating multiple patients in the same peaceful room for a smaller fee).[12] Acupuncture is also offered in some hospitals; ask your care team if the service is available while you are hospitalized. Some cancer programs offer acupuncture and other traditional treatments as complementary therapy.

I was surprised how much [acupuncture] helped with my allergies and pain. It also improved my anxiety. It felt like a good reset to my nervous system. I had always had abdominal pain that Western medicine couldn't address. The Western understanding of our nerves and our electrical system seemed limited and reductionist. The Eastern version that acupuncture offered made more sense. It gave me a broader sense of being connected. It also improved my pain.

I have continued acupuncture for the last nine years because I find it sooth-ing. I feel like it alleviates a lot of stagnation I feel in my body. I keep it in my handbook of things I like to do to keep my body working well.

East Asian Medicine

East Asian medicine looks at the body differently than Western medicine. In Western medicine the body is the macrocosm and all the components of cells and DNA are the microcosm, whereas in Chinese medicine the body is the microcosm and everything we come into contact with during our entire life is the macrocosm. Because everything we come into contact [with] affects our health.

—Jennifer Ashby, DAOM, L.Ac., integrative East Asian medicine doctor

East Asian medicine (EAM) includes medicine and medical practices from throughout Asia. EAM includes traditional Chinese medicine (TCM), a sys-tem of medical care that originated in China and is based in the philoso-phy of Taoism. Encompassing a wide range of medical practices, including mind-body work, exercise, herbal medicine, and nutrition, EAM is based on returning the body from a state of unbalance to a state of homeostasis, or balanced physiology.

In EAM, illness comes from a lack of balance. Many people with long illness resonate deeply with this philosophy. Treatment centers on regain-ing balance and harmony by understanding the flow of energy through the body (qi) and balancing organ systems using Eastern philosophies of the body and universe (for example, yin and yang). During a visit with an EAM practitioner, you will be asked detailed questions about your body and life aimed at understanding patterns of unbalance in your body. Your pulses, tongue, and complexion will be examined. Seeing an EAM practitioner can be a different type of experience for someone with a long illness, who may be used to feeling their body fragmented by medical specialties, or hearing small complaints invalidated.

Dr. Ashby explains that "the goal is to find the origins of the insult that caused the illness in your body. A lot of my patients will say to me, 'I just want my life back.' And in a very appropriate way I say, 'No, you don't.' Because whatever that life was before created enough of an imbalance for disease to thrive."

EXERCISE

STRETCHES TO MOVE QI IN YOUR BODY

Our channels of qi (energy) start or end in the hands and feet. When we are tense, stressed, sick, or anxious, we close or even clench our hands and feel ungrounded. Here is an exercise you can try to open up your hands and feet to allow your energy to flow. If parts of this exercise feel uncomfortable or painful, stop. Imagining the movements of your hands and feet and the movement of qi also provides a benefit. You can do this exercise on yourself, or have someone else do the exercise on you.

Place your hands in a prayer position at your chest level, fingers pointed toward the sky. Push your palms against each other. Then bring the hands in prayer down toward your belly button to stretch the tendons in your wrists.

Now reverse the direction of your hands, so that the backs of your hands are pressed firmly together with the fingers pointed toward the ground in reverse prayer position. Bring your hands up toward your nose, as if someone were pulling up on your arms, until you feel a stretch in your wrists and forearms.

Finger stretches: Wrap your right hand around your left pointer finger and gently pull. At the end of the pull, pull in the up direction at the tip of the finger, to make sure the qi is not stagnant and continues to flow rather than pooling at the end of the finger. Wrap and pull each finger on your left hand. Then swap hands. If you hear a little pop, that's okay. Next, going finger by finger, push each finger back toward your hand to get a stretch (extension).

Twisting: *Twisting improves blood flow and qi and is easier if someone else does this to you. That person will wrap their hands around your forearm and twist one hand to the right and the other to the left, as though gently wringing out a wet rag. They will move up your arm and then down to your fingertips, twisting one finger at a time. They should always end on an up-twist to keep the qi flowing.*

Foot stretches: *If you do not have someone to stretch your toes and feet for you, you can push against the floor. For floor stretches, sit down on the floor with the balls of your feet on the floor. Lift and lower your foot. To stretch the front of the foot while sitting in a chair, roll your foot over your toes so that your toes almost touch the bottoms of your feet. Continue to roll your foot forward to get a stretch in front of your ankle.*

Ayurveda

Ayurvedic medicine, developed thousands of years ago in India, is a holistic approach to health that uses products, exercise, diet, and lifestyle to maintain and improve health. It can be particularly useful in long illness because it is a form of medicine that sees the mind and body as connected and that uses many modalities of healing.

Ayurveda translates to "knowledge of life." If you practice yoga, you already have some knowledge of Ayurveda, as they are related. Like East Asian medicine, Ayurveda is based on the idea that disease comes from imbalance or stress, but Ayurvedic philosophy focuses on imbalances in a person's enlightened awareness of themselves and the world (consciousness). The goal of treatments is to regain balance between the body, mind, spirit, and environment, focusing on *prana*, the life force that flows through us (similar to qi in East Asian medicine).

Doshas are energetic forces of nature that make up our constitution. Everyone is born with a mixture of the three doshas: *pitta, kapha,* and *vata.* Over time, because of your experiences, a particular dosha or doshas might dominate. When dosha levels are in excess in your body, you can become ill.

Dosha	Specific Energy	Constitutive Elements	Results of Excess
Pitta	Transformation	Fire and water	Anger, jealousy, inflammation, heartburn, diarrhea, migraines, rashes, bruises, hunger, insomnia
Kapha	Cohesiveness	Earth and water	Greed, lack of motivation, feeling of heaviness, excessive sleep, depression, water retention, resistance to change
Vata	Creativity, connection	Air and space	Anxiety, fear, constipation, dry skin, insomnia, tremors

Ayurvedic treatment usually includes internal purification (cleansing) paired with a strict diet, herbs, yoga, meditation, and massage. Many of the cleansing, massage, and skin treatments have become popularized recently, as they are healing to skin and relaxing. Many Ayurvedic herbs and spices also have gained attention over the last several decades, as they have been found to have anti-inflammatory and antioxidant properties. Golden milk lattes, for example, have roots in Ayurveda.

Anti-Inflammatory Ayurvedic Spices and Herbs	Properties
Ashwagandha	Helps manage stress by reducing cortisol; helpful for anxiety symptoms
Boswellia	Aids in digestion and helps breathing in patients with asthma
Cumin	Helps with digestion of fats; eat when bloated or having abdominal pain
Licorice root	Helpful with bloating and heartburn
Turmeric	Curcumin is the active compound that, when ingested with black pepper, provides antioxidant and anti-inflammatory benefits. Research suggests that it increases blood flow and improves depression and cognition. Large amounts must be ingested to get benefits, however, and black pepper can be upsetting to the GI tract. Try adding some turmeric to your diet.

Despite its widespread use as primary medical care in India and nearby areas, there have been few well-designed research trials on Ayurvedic medicine practices. There is no licensing or accreditation for these practitioners in most countries. To find a good practitioner, you need to do your research. In the United States, a good place to start is the National Ayurvedic Medical Association (ayurvedanama.org). If you are not in the United States, check with the national Ayurvedic association in your country, most of which have a list of practitioners registered with their organization.

Traditional Products and Treatments

Medications, teas, tinctures, pills, and potions prescribed by traditional practitioners vary greatly in reliability and safety. Be sure to work with a practitioner you trust, ask for an ingredient list, and ask for information about the supplies of ingredients. Even governmentally tested and regulated medication can be contaminated or adulterated. Being "traditional" or "natural" does not make it safe. Arsenic, lead, and mercury are all "natural" and sometimes contaminate preparations of traditional ingredients. However, they are all toxins that should not be ingested. (See Chapter 21 on natural products and supplements.)

Some preparations might be repurposed conventional medicine, such as the anti-inflammatory medications (like steroids or nonsteroidal anti-inflammatories) that may be added to herbs. This can be harmful for people with different medical conditions, and you may unintentionally take unsafe levels of these medications, especially if you are taking them regularly. If your practitioner doesn't want to share information about the safety of their products, it's not worth your time. There is no magic potion or cure that keeps its source or ingredients secret. When you have a long illness, your money, time, and patience are already stretched a bit thin. You can avoid dealing with side effects and possible toxin exposure with a little research and clear communication with your practitioners. To avoid any contraindications, be sure to inform your traditional medicine practitioners of any medications you are taking and inform your conventional practitioners of any additional products or supplements you are considering taking.

Choosing a Traditional Medicine Practitioner

The more years of experience a practitioner has, the more likely they are to be able to help you manage a complex issue. As with all relationships with those on your medical team, it is important that you like your practitioner. According to Dr. Ashby, "This is a long-term relationship that you are going to return to over the years as problems flare up. It's someone you want to be really comfortable with."

Traditional medicine practitioners are being integrated into many major medical centers, working alongside biomedically trained health care teams. Check with your health care team to see if they can refer you to traditional medicine practitioners in your health care system. You can also use our resources section.

CHAPTER 21

Natural Products and Supplements

I have spent hundreds of dollars on supplements. At one point, I was seeing someone who had me on a different supplement every week. It was a lot of money and made me feel bad when they didn't work. I had to do my own research and find integrative doctors who knew about supplements. Now I'm on just a few that I know work. In times of stress, I add on one or two more. I don't stay on anything I don't think is helping, and I reevaluate every few months.

What You Will Learn in This Chapter:

- An overview of the use of supplements and natural products in long illness
- How to pick a product that is safe and regulated
- An exploration of stress-regulating adaptogens

There is rarely a single medication that addresses all the symptoms of a long illness. Pharmaceutical medicines fall short. And even when they help to control symptoms, many people experience intolerable side effects from them. Natural products are an important part of the treatment plan for many people with long illness. We use supplements and natural products every day in our clinic, but we approach them with the same rigor we bring to our biomedicines.

If you have googled your symptoms, you might have noticed the ads popping up for pills and potions that will fix you. Your friends might swear that supplement X changed their symptoms. Your cabinets might be full of brain fog supplements recommended by friends, practitioners, and sales-people. But what should you actually be taking? How do you know what works best for your condition—and what might be a waste of money? How do you know if what you are taking is safe? This chapter will unpack some of the mysteries and questions about supplements for long illness.

About 20 percent of Americans take at least one supplement or natural product daily. A *natural product* is a chemical or substance made by a living organism that can be used to prevent or treat disease or enhance performance or experience. These substances can be harvested from nature directly or made synthetically in labs. Natural products serve as a great resource for drug discovery. Some of the most common drugs used in conventional medicine are synthetic, more potent versions of natural products, such as hormones, vitamins, plant antioxidants, breast milk, cobra venom, poppy plants, and willow bark.

Natural products are limited by their bioavailability, that is, by how much of the active ingredient can get into the blood. As more research is conducted on natural products, the pharmacological potential of these compounds will be clarified and refined. However, most natural products, including supplements, are not subject to the same level of scrutiny as pharmaceutical drugs, and active ingredient levels and their quality vary widely between different products.

Supplements are any substance taken in addition to dietary intake that is intended to provide nutrients or increase the ability of the body to absorb or utilize nutrients. Examples include vitamins, minerals, herbs, amino acids (parts of protein), fatty acids, and fiber. Supplements often include or are a natural product.

In the United States, these products must carry a clear label stating that natural products are not sold by regulated pharmaceutical companies as a drug to prevent or treat disease. The idea that something "natural" can help their disease is appealing to many, but because these products are less regulated, they can have a number of issues. First, being natural doesn't necessarily mean something is safe. Second, in a market with less regulation of a product, not everyone is going to sell the best or safest product. So how do you know which ones to buy?

When you walk into any grocery store in the United States these days, you are usually greeted by at least one wall of supplements. Navigating all the flashy packaging and health claims is overwhelming. Your prescriber recommends magnesium, but what kind? What do you need to know when picking a natural product or supplement?

Is What You're Buying Safe?

Dietary supplements send thousands of people to the emergency room every year in the United States alone. It is important to include your health care team in any decisions you make to take supplements and to do your research. Having a long illness requires that you be a bit more thoughtful about what goes into your body, including supplements.

Prescription drug side effects and adverse events are tracked by the US Food and Drug Administration (FDA). The close surveillance of drugs allows for them to be quickly taken off the market and for consumers to be notified if dangerous reactions to these products are discovered. Supplements, which are not regulated by the FDA, are not subject to such surveillance.

That said, makers of natural products can apply for multiple seals of approval guaranteeing that the product is as advertised on the label. A product that doesn't have every seal of approval is not necessarily unsafe.

Ingredient and Product Verifications

Good Manufacturing Practice (GMP): The GMP verification confirms that the ingredients, the final product, and the manufacturing facility have been inspected for contamination, adulteration, and sanitation. The seal says "Certified GMP," "FDA Approved Facility," or "CGMP Inspected Facility."

Third-party verification: The NSF seal (formerly the National Sanitation Foundation) and USP (United States Pharmacopeial Convention) seal come from third-party verification services paid by manufacturers of supplements to monitor the quality of their ingredients and products. The FDA does not have the bandwidth to test all the supplements that exist, so these labels, granted after a process similar to the FDA's, can provide peace of mind for the consumer.

Production and Manufacturing Verification

USDA Organic: This seal tells you that the supplement you are buying has been created without unapproved chemicals, including herbicides, pesticides, or antibiotics, genetically modified organisms, and sewage.

Non-GMO Project Verified: A supplement earns this seal when every step in the production of the supplement has been tested and confirmed as free of genetically modified organisms.

Fair Trade Certified: This seal ensures that all of the steps in the production of the supplement were completed in a way that improved lives where they were made and protected the environment.

ConsumerLab.com independently tests products to make sure that the contents match the description. For an annual membership fee, it makes available reviews and recommendations of brands for the most commonly used supplements. We use this website in our clinical practice. Ideally, you won't have to purchase a membership because a member of your health care team will have one. But if you frequently purchase supplements, it may be worth the investment. (Consider sharing a membership with a friend.)

Can Supplements Interfere with Other Medications You're Taking?

Supplements may interact with your medications in such a way as to make them more potent or less effective. When you get a prescription, your practitioner and your pharmacist should both check to ensure that the prescribed medication will not interact adversely with the medications you already take (contraindications). That is why it is important to tell all your practitioners about all the medication you take. You can also take a look for yourself on the Natural Medicines Comprehensive Database.[13] This database is a good resource for looking up the effectiveness of natural medicine products for various conditions, their interactions with drugs, and other educational information.

As natural products and supplements have become more popular while remaining minimally regulated, multiple exposés on their harms have been published. Although there is some truth to these stories, using the guidelines here, and with the help of your care team, you can find safe and reliable products.

What Are Adaptogens?

Adaptogens are natural products that help the body resist the effects of stress. If taken regularly, they may train your body to handle stress itself. Since long illness is inherently stressful, adaptogens are often incorporated into a treatment plan for long illness. These substances are roots, herbs, or the fruit of plants, and some derive from mushrooms (fungus). You might have seen them added to your favorite coffee drinks, smoothies, and teas or sold as supplements.

Adaptogens have many health benefits, including protecting your nerve cells, fighting fatigue, enhancing your immune system, reducing anxiety and depression, giving you energy, improving your sleep, and enhancing your brain performance. Each adaptogen has its own unique effect. Their effect on your stress level comes from their interaction with chemicals that are part of your stress response pathway (such as cortisol and nitric oxide). Many adaptogens have been used in traditional medicine for centuries.

One of the defining characteristics of adaptogens is their nontoxicity at the doses recommended for stress resistance. Taken this way, they are generally not harmful, although people who are sensitive to certain adaptogenic chemicals should start slowly and listen to their body. For example, some people are very sensitive to anything that might stimulate their nervous system, so taking ginseng or rhodiola might be too activating for them. Others might be able to tolerate higher doses without feeling any stimulating effect. Although current data support the use of many of these substances, you should be wary of companies that claim to offer adaptogens, as they are even less regulated than supplements. It is important to talk to a knowledgeable practitioner about an adaptogen that might be useful for you and about where to find a reliable source.

With adaptogens, just as with other supplements, we stick to the rules of adding one at a time, starting low (dose), and going slow. Maybe ashwagandha is what will help you deal with stress, but if you add it in with other new chemicals, you might not see its effect, or you might not know which supplement you ingested seemed to change your symptoms, for better or worse.

Do any of the following adaptogens look familiar to you? Have you tried any of them in the past or do you currently take them? What has worked for you? Do you see any here that interest you?

Adaptogen	Beneficial Effects
Ashwagandha root	Reduces long-term stress, protects against stress and anxiety, lowers cortisol level
Astragalus root	Eases fatigue and inflammation in asthma and allergies
Bacopa herb	Reduces inflammation, improves memory
Cordyceps fungus	Reduces stress, balances hormones, reduces cravings for sugar, improves physical performance
Curcumin (turmeric root)	Reduces inflammation, balances stress
Eleutherococcus root (Siberian ginseng)	Reduces short-term stress and anxiety, boosts immune system, increases energy, improves physical performance, helps with menopausal symptoms and osteoporosis
Ginseng root (American or Asian)	Lessens long-term stress, boosts immune system, reduces inflammation, improves memory
Holy basil (contains calcium, zinc, iron, and vitamins A and C)	Lowers stress levels, decreases anxiety, reduces inflammation
Licorice root	Boosts endurance, increases energy, makes you lose water (diuretic)
Maca root (contains vitamin C, copper, zinc, iron, and calcium)	Boosts mood, increases energy, supports women's hormonal issues (including PMS, menopause, and hot flashes)

Reishi fungus	Boosts immune system, relieves stress
Rhodiola root	Reduces short-term stress and anxiety, increases energy, improves physical performance, improves memory
Schisandra berries	Reduces short-term stress and anxiety, protects brain cells, boosts memory and cognitive function, improves liver function, helps with GI issues

EXERCISE

TRYING AN ADAPTOGEN

First, let your health care team know that you are going to try an adaptogen for a week. Pick an adaptogen that you think might be helpful for you. Do your research and see if it's a good fit. Plan to try it at a time when little else is going on. Taking the adaptogen can be as simple as adding it to your foods or drinking a tea infused with it.

After taking the adaptogen for a week, check in with yourself:

Do you feel any changes in your body?

Do you feel as though stress affected you differently this past week?

Did you feel the effects that are claimed to be associated with the adaptogen?

Would you find this adaptogen useful in the future when you are stressed out or know that you're going to be under more stress?

What Is Homeopathy? Is It a Natural Product?

Technically yes, since homeopathy uses tiny amounts of natural substances (like plants and minerals). But homeopathy is actually an entire medical system based on the idea that "like cures like": the belief that substances that bring on symptoms in us when we take them in large amounts can cure those symptoms when given in small amounts. In homeopathy, substances are diluted in water or some other substance until, as often happens, they are no longer detectable. Scientific studies have shown no difference between any homeopathic preparation and a placebo, and they do not support a role for the homeopathic model of care in curing disease.

Homeopathy is not a part of our medical practices because there just isn't the evidence to support its use. Some people, however, have described its benefits. We humbly acknowledge that some things work in ways that research might not yet be able to quantify.

What if Your Practitioner Doesn't Know About the Natural Product You Want to Try?

Practitioners might not have specific knowledge about what you are interested in taking, but they spent years learning how to find high-quality information. Show them what you have found and ask if they can provide you with more information or with their opinion based on experience. It's okay to ask more than one practitioner about a medication if you are on the fence about taking it. Supplements range from being strongly evidence-based to untested and even harmful in some conditions, so it is useful to involve your practitioners in this discussion. Supplements also can interact with medications you are already taking, so make sure to check with your team before starting anything new. Pharmacists can also be a good resource, as they are the experts in medication interactions. Another good place to start narrowing the list of natural products and supplements you're interested in is to ask your friends who also have a long illness about their experiences with natural products and about brands they might recommend.

How Do You Decide Whether You Should Take a Natural Product?

We recommend asking yourself these questions:

> Is this product recommended for your condition or situation? For example, for people on steroids, vitamin D and calcium are recommended. Think about cost. Is this product covered by your insurance? If not, can you use your health savings account or flex spending account to pay for it? How much would it cost per month if you take the recommended dose? Can you afford it? Is there a way to get it covered by a

charity program from the manufacturer or a charity care fund? Some manufacturers will give you cost-reduced supplements if you fill out forms on their websites and get supporting notes from a practitioner.

Are there common side effects from this supplement? Are these symptoms you already deal with that might get worse? How could you minimize the side effects? (For example, you might take the supplement with food to avoid nausea, or drink more water to prevent headache.)

Are there possible interactions between the supplement and the medications you already take? Who can you talk to about ways to mitigate an interaction?

We recommend that you make a list of the pros and cons of taking the natural product or supplement you are considering. Then try it out for a few weeks or months, one supplement at a time, unless your care team recommends starting multiple supplements at once. Pay attention to whether the supplement changes how you feel. If you aren't sure, try stopping it for a few months to see if you feel any different. Of course, this advice does not apply to supplements that prevent disease or are backed by strong evidence. Continue to check in with your health care team, illness community, and yourself to think about whether you should add or drop a natural product or supplement, since you might need it only at different times of your illness or symptoms. You will become an expert in what works best for you.

CHAPTER 22

Resilience and Goals

Resilience is letting me feel my feels: sometimes I would cry and sometimes I would scream, and sometimes I would throw things, and sometimes I would tell the nurse to get the fuck out of my room. Sometimes you have to acknowledge the fact that you have limits; part of being resilient is realizing this is something that you're just not able to do right now. It's also letting other people in. So it can be kind of scary to think, "I'm going to tell someone exactly what this is like." But part of being resilient is letting someone in and letting someone know, "Sometimes my life really sucks."

What You Will Learn in This Chapter:

- What resilience means in long illness
- How to identify what depletes your resilience and what boosts it
- Gentle strategies to move toward goals that align with vitality, even in the face of illness

Long illnesses wax and wane. There are times when your symptoms may be so severe that just making it through the day takes everything you've got. Today may be a day when brushing your teeth and feeding yourself is the best you can do. That's okay. This chapter isn't written to make you feel bad for not being able to do things you want to be doing but can't. Long illness is hard enough without that kind of messaging.

People with a long illness sometimes internalize a message that they are fragile or lack endurance, and this message is often conveyed, unfortunately, by our medical system. Some practitioners get frustrated when they're not able to solve a problem, and they project the blame onto their patients. This message can also come at home from friends and family when *they mistake struggle for weakness.*

Being considered fragile and lacking in endurance isn't fair to you, and in our experience it just isn't true of people with a long illness. You aren't weak because you struggle—in fact, the opposite is true. Your challenges have made you stronger and more resilient. You can learn how to see that strength and resilience.

Let's start by understanding resilience. Resilience is not necessarily acceptance. Rather, it is that part of you that whispers, *Keep going!* when every other part of you says you can't. Resilience can be lessened or strengthened by your relationships, life experience, health, and childhood. You can learn how to be resilient and how to improve it. In fact, our guess is that you are already part of the way there.

Did a Childhood Full of Adverse Events Make You Less Resilient?

No. Many people experience significant stressors in childhood. Roughly 60 percent of people experience a severe trauma, but only a small percentage experience prolonged stress disorders (like PTSD). Although childhood trauma is a risk factor for developing stress-related illness as an adult, you can modify this risk factor by taking action to increase your resiliency pathways and strengthen your coping skills.

Traumatic childhood events can live on in our reactions to everyday stressors. In the midst of a current experience, you may relive a memory of past trauma at the same time. Understanding how your experiences impact your response to stress is the first step to changing that response.

Bolstering Resilience

Bolstering your resilience will help with every aspect of your healing. Sometimes we don't realize when something or someone is depleting our ability to persist in the face of challenges. In medical studies, there is good support for using CBT and mindfulness to increase resilience, and these may work for you. But everyone's resilience has a unique blend of ingredients. Let's add more to your resiliency tool kit.

Imagine that resilience is like a bank account. What takes money out? What puts money in?

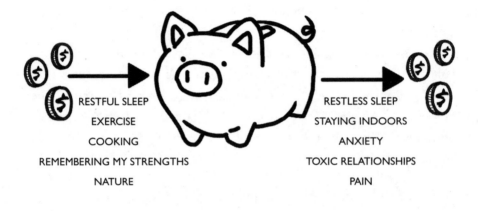

RESTFUL SLEEP
EXERCISE
COOKING
REMEMBERING MY STRENGTHS
NATURE

RESTLESS SLEEP
STAYING INDOORS
ANXIETY
TOXIC RELATIONSHIPS
PAIN

Journaling

YOUR RESILIENCY BANK ACCOUNT

Step 1: Read each word in the list on page 305 of common things that strengthen or deplete resilience. Sit with each word and ask yourself: Does this give me energy, does it take energy away, or is it neutral? If it is something not relevant to you, ignore it.

Step 2: In your journal, create three columns, one titled "Strengthening," one titled "Depleting," and one titled "Neutral." Copy each word in the list into the column that corresponds to your feelings about it.

Step 3: Look at your "Strengthening" list. Are there more of these activities or practices you could incorporate into your day? What about what you've copied into the "Depleting" column? How can you avoid some of the things in your life that drain you?

Relationships	Diet	Engagement	
Family	Energy-promoting foods	Volunteer work	
Partner	Ultra-processed foods	Paid work	
Healthy friendships	Anti-inflammatory foods	Hobbies	
Invalidating friendships	Cooking	Making art	
One-sided relationships	Takeout	Making music	
Toxic relationships		Community work	
Making new friends		Sense of purpose	
Self-Care	**Well-Being**	**Exercise**	
Psychotherapy	Depression	Sitting around all day	
Journaling	Anxiety	Movement lying down	
Mindfulness	Past trauma	Movement while seated	
Meditation	Feeling misunderstood	Light housework	
Baths/showers	Feeling understood	Light errands	
Massage	Peaceful moments	Cleaning	
Grooming	Bottling emotions	Jogging/running	
Cleaning	People pleasing	Swimming	
Staying indoors	Pain	Yoga/Pilates	
Music	Restful sleep	Weight lifting	
TV/movies	Restless sleep	Tai chi	
Reading	Remembering personal		
Going outside	strengths		
Being in nature			

Journaling

CELEBRATE YOUR BRAVERY

Write about a time when you felt brave as you overcame an obstacle. If it's hard to remember how you felt, try recounting the incident from the perspective of a friend or family member. What story would they share about your bravery?

EXERCISE

MINDFULNESS: GIVE YOUR RESILIENCE WINGS

By making space in your mind, you can give your resilience a chance to build. Over the next few minutes, use the inhale of your breath to amplify and draw in your strength. On the exhale, gently acknowledge any parts of yourself that feel insecure and invite those parts to join with your strength.

Set a ten-minute timer and focus on your breath.

Take a moment to center yourself. Take five breaths.

On the inhale, feel your strength, feel your grit, feel the part or parts of yourself that persist.

As you exhale, gently acknowledge any parts of yourself that feel scared, that feel alone, that feel guilt, shame, or fear.

On your next inhale, invite these parts to join with your strength, to build your strength, to feel your inherent and expansive worth.

Repeat this cycle. On the inhale, try to focus on your resilience, strength, and fortitude. On the exhale, identify any parts of yourself that feel brittle, scared, or alone. On the following inhale, invite these parts to join with your strength.

Upon closing, take a moment to feel your strength radiating in and through you. Reflect on all of what this strength has done for you. Continue to invite parts of yourself that are scared or alone to join with this strength.

End with a deep gratitude for yourself, your imperfectly perfect self. You are strong. You are enough.

Small Changes Build Momentum: Goal Setting and Long Illness

An object in motion remains in motion. An object at rest remains at rest.
—Newton's First Law of Motion

Change is hard, even for people not living with the complexities of long illness. But without the progress that only comes from change, we feel stuck and our self-esteem can take a hit. It is also challenging when our goals or visions for ourselves get derailed by ill health.

With long illnesses, there is an ebb and flow of setbacks and steps forward. Relapses may be the body's way of trying to heal itself. When a knot isn't tied right, you have to untie it before you can retie it. We like the traditional medicine perspective that a relapse is a time when the body is communicating something more that it needs. At the very least, these frustrating periods of regression can encourage you to change habits and pick up new tools.

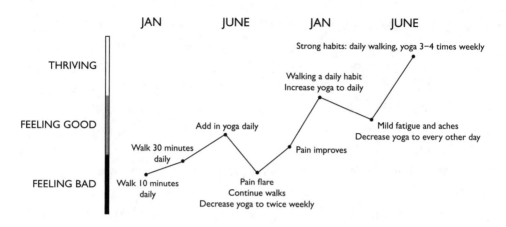

The chart here shows the typical pattern we see in people when they adopt new health behaviors. In it, a person with fibromyalgia is starting to exercise. Their progress is anything but a straight line, but they manage to make big changes by gathering momentum from small changes. They listen to their body. They continue to take small steps forward, even after setbacks.

You may not feel ready to make changes. Perhaps this moment is too painful a time to be pushing any further. That's okay. *You are reading this book, and that means you are considering something new.* Seeds are being planted for the future. You can allow a little more time before the growth begins.

> *When I am sick, I can get overwhelmed with the big picture. What I have found helpful is to get everything onto paper, where I can see what's going on. Then I break down tasks into smaller and smaller chunks. When I'm not in top shape, breaking things down into smaller bits makes it so that I can keep moving. Any progress is good progress. It doesn't have to be perfect progress to be good progress. So that way you can keep moving forward, even when you're not in ideal condition.*

When you're ready to set some goals, keep the following in mind:

Set SMART goals. It is important that your goals are your own, not what someone else thinks you need. Once you have a goal in mind, you can use CBT to help you craft a goal that is the most achievable. We use the following mnemonic: set SMART (Specific, Measurable, Attainable, Relevant, and Time-Based) goals.

Specific: Your goal should be specific and narrow. Don't overwhelm yourself with a goal that is too big. How do you climb Mount Everest? One step at a time.

Measurable: Ask yourself how you will measure your progress to your goal.

Attainable: Make sure your goal is realistic for you and your health.

Relevant: The goal should be important to *you*.

Time-Based: Set a realistic time line for achieving your goal.

Here are some examples of SMART goals:

I will walk one mile within three months. I will start today by walking for ten minutes.

I will meditate for ten minutes per day for two weeks.

Within one week I will reach out to three psychotherapists who contract with my insurance.

Evaluate your barriers. Listen to the struggle you feel when you're considering a change. Be mindful of your resistance. Once you are aware of an internal barrier, try practicing the skills you learned in previous chapters.

Try to identify your resistance. Examples of internal barriers include stinking thinking (thoughts like "what's the point" or "I am never getting better"), fear of changing your routine, fear of failure, fatigue, fear of the effect on relationships, and low motivation. For example, if stinking thinking is a barrier, try practicing the skills we practiced earlier (described in Chapter 12).

Examples of external barriers include finances, transportation, weather, limited time, and child care. Although many external barriers can't be changed, or at least not quickly, it can be useful to get them down on paper to help you understand the current landscape. With brainstorming, you may discover places where external barriers can be shifted slightly to make more room for your goals.

Move toward your goals but be flexible about the outcome. For example, Lisa has a goal of walking two miles within six months. She walks four times per week. Because of pain and fatigue, she is not able to walk two miles, even after diligent practice. But she can walk a mile and a half. Being able to walk this distance is still moving toward her goal, even if the outcome looks different.

A note on procrastination: *procrastination is a compromise.* By putting something off, your mind accomplishes two things: it prevents you from experiencing the discomfort of change, and it shields you from the disappointment of abandoning a goal. But the anxiety it produces is almost always worse than the potential discomfort and disappointment combined! Try to be mindful of how much anxiety your procrastination generates. Try taking just a small step. That's a better compromise than procrastination!

Look for *progress, not perfection.* Perfect isn't the goal. Studies have shown us that it takes two to three months for a new behavior to become a consistent habit. Listen closely to your body and create goals that are realistic and healthy. You are a human being, *not* a human doing.

Journaling

VITALITY

> If there is one thing you could change this week that could move you toward vitality, what would it be? Why?
>
> Write out one goal you can try today or this week. Try to use the SMART guidelines above to craft your goal.
>
> What will your life look like when you make this change?
>
> What barriers do you see to accomplishing this goal? What strengths can you use to help you accomplish this goal?

CHAPTER 23

Your Story Is Powerful

In This Chapter You Will:

- Learn about narrative medicine, a powerful tool for self-healing in long illness
- Understand how narrative medicine shifts the body and brain
- Reflect on and deepen your understanding of your experiences by creating a Life Tree

Writing has been a way that I reconnected with my own voice. I got to write in a way that was completely unfiltered and only for me. More has revealed itself to me as I keep writing. I don't feel confused anymore. I can go slower now. I know that there is still more to uncover, but this simple tool has reduced my pain and anxiety.

Your story is uniquely yours and meaningful. But when you are sick, it might not feel that way. Maybe in your illness you have not been heard, seen, or validated. Maybe you have been told how to feel and think. Maybe you thought there was a right way to be sick. But you do not have to fit a mold. Your experience is real.

Narrative practice is a self-exploration tool that works like some forms of therapy to help you understand your own mind. It includes journaling and writing to help your brain explore thoughts it isn't used to.

Think about your story: your childhood, key events in your life, everything that explains who you are and what's important to you. Reclaiming your story can be important to healing. Truth is powerful. Reflecting on the past can change the present.

Memories and the Brain

Memories and experiences are stored in your brain. Without you knowing it, some of your memories are still being lived in this moment, especially traumatic memories and experiences that feel unaddressed. Whether consciously or not, *you are living not only your current experience but your past experiences as well.* A part of your brain remembers your painful experiences and is working hard to protect you against future hurt. If the memory is traumatic and unaddressed, it may still be causing you pain, even though you aren't consciously aware of it.

The mind can't always tell the difference between a past threat and a current threat. Your brain crafts defense mechanisms to protect you from painful memories and the prospect of future hurt. There are many defense mechanisms, including anxiety and dissociation. Each of these defenses serves a purpose! Anxiety keeps you on the lookout for danger. Dissociation is your mind trying to disconnect you from something that could hurt you.

With many defense mechanisms, the cure can be worse than the disease. If pieces of your history are traumatic and undigested, your brain may use these mechanisms *all the time*, instead of only as needed. An unrelenting defense mechanism is like wearing a suit of armor 24/7. Imagine watching TV or going to the beach in a full suit of armor. The mental energy that a constant defense mechanism requires could be spent in other places. When your own brain is using that energy to protect you, it's not available to be creative or relax.

Narrative Medicine for Long Illness

Some of our patients with a long illness had a traumatic experience early in life. Even if you didn't have traumatic experiences before you became sick, a change in your identity, a feeling of being invalidated, unrelenting symptoms, and other medical experiences can be traumatic. Unaddressed trauma and memories can lead to an overactivation of the fight-or-flight sympathetic nervous system. As we learned in Chapter 1, activation of this system can affect every organ of the body. We think that an overactive sympathetic nervous system is a big part of the body dysfunction we see in long illness. While undigested emotional trauma is not exclusively responsible, we know that it can contribute to a revving of the engine of your fight-or-flight nervous system.

How Does Writing Your Story Work?

Solely focusing on the story of today is like examining one brushstroke of a painting. Writing out your stories of your life gives you a chance to take a step back, look at the whole painting, and develop perspective.

Journaling is an effective treatment for conditions like post-traumatic stress disorder. Writing about our memories can transform them, bringing about powerful changes when they hit the page. Something about that memory can start to shift. Journaling lets you be seen and heard by *you* and gives you a chance to reconnect with yourself. While unearthing your story can be uncomfortable, positive feelings almost always follow. At the end of the exercises described here, our patients have said they felt lighter, more centered and empowered, and more whole.

How to Start Writing

Many people who start with our exercise and journaling prompts feel driven to write more. A lot of threads came together to weave the tapestry of you. Pull at one thread at a time and see what else is connected to it. Start writing whenever you are ready. This isn't a command (many of our patients are so hard on themselves that any suggestion feels like that!), but an invitation.

A few things to keep in mind:

If it isn't time for you to write yet, consider at least reading the exercises here. Your brain may start to process your story even if you aren't writing.

Your mind may take you to the places that need healing the most, whether it's trauma, painful memories, or shame. If these uncomfortable sensations arise, try to write about them if you feel yourself pulled in that direction. *The more you connect your feelings to memories, the more healing the writing can be.* But be gentle with yourself. Take breaks if you need them. If you start to feel unsafe, activated, or as though this process is too intense, you can stop at any time. Bring yourself back to the present moment. Try the senses exercise on page 185 to bring yourself back to your current space or take some time outdoors. Remember to keep breathing, because deep breaths recruit your nervous system to help you return to the present moment.

If you end up in a space that feels overwhelming, reach out for help from a trusted adviser, medical team member, therapist, or friend. Try to remember that even though *you are living a memory*, that memory is not your reality in the present moment. Writing down your story can bring up uncomfortable feelings and emotions, but it shouldn't be destabilizing or retraumatizing. If it feels like it is, it may be better to pursue journaling with a mental health professional walking alongside you for support.

For many people, some memories are clear and some are fuzzier. Pieces of yourself can scatter after a trauma. And the experience of a long illness is traumatic. If trauma or long illness has happened to you, it is not your fault. Your mind may feel like it has dammed up those tender memories with rocks. Writing can feel like hard work. You are picking up those rocks and looking underneath them. By doing this hard work, you will come to know yourself again.

When memories or emotions feel stuck, don't strain to bring them out. When you are relaxed and in the flow, they may reappear. Listen to your thoughts. Let them guide you.

We trust your recollection of your own memories. Many of our patients have experienced invalidation from other people ("you don't look sick"). Write what is true for you. We believe you.

Some people experience even deeper healing when they read what they have written to a therapist or trusted friend. You can choose to do this or not. You get to decide if it feels right to share your story, and who will have the privilege of learning about your journey.

Journaling

LIFE TREE

If you are ready to write your story, go write! For everyone else, let's start by developing your Life Tree. Once you have labeled your tree, you can move on to the journaling prompts, which will help you start freely describing your experiences.

We recommend starting at the roots and answering the questions from the bottom up. If you need more space, you can draw your own tree in your journal or use the blank tree in Appendix F on page 329. On the next page, you will see an example of a Life Tree filled out by a person living with long illness.

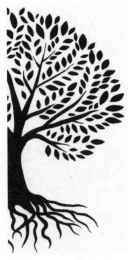

Leaves What does your life look like today?
Important people, hobbies, career, hopes, dreams

Branches What roles or experiences helped define you?
Big events, life roles

Trunk Who did you grow into?
Skills, abilities, talents, values

Roots Where do you come from?
Family, culture, childhood experiences and hobbies

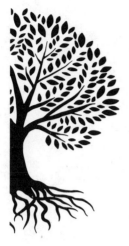

Leaves What does your life look like today?
Important people, hobbies, obligations, career, hopes, dreams

Want children	Painting	Dogs	Design	Long walks
Medical appointments	Dating	Friends	Student loans	Anxiety

Branches What roles or experiences helped define you?
Big events, life roles

College	Car accident
Illness	Art

Trunk Who did you grow into?
Skills, abilities, talents, values

Artist	Adaptable	Generous	Funny
Talented	People pleasing	Intuitive	Smart

Roots Where do you come from?
Family, culture, childhood experiences and hobbies

Love nature	Reading	Loving grandma	Loved school	Mexican food
Volleyball	Money issues	Distracted mom	Trauma	Moved a lot

TIPS

- As you fill in your tree, include any memories or experiences that come to mind. Some may bring you joy, and others may bring discomfort or pain, but including both the darkness and the light in your life can help you write the most complete story.
- Write anywhere. Allow the tree to be messy.
- Don't get too caught up with organization! Allow your creativity and healing mind to take the lead.
- When your inner critic emerges, simply observe it. A part of you is probably scared, and this is the way that part is trying to manage this fear. You are safe in this moment of reclaiming your memories.
- The space in the journal here may not be enough. Use a notebook or type on your computer. Feel free to draw your own tree.

Journaling

EXPLORING YOUR TREE

Write more about one or more of the roots of your life.

Write more about one or more of the branches of your life.

Where is your mind taking you next? Write freely about any experience or memory.

Conclusion

Long Ending

I try to use as many tools as I can, but sometimes I get taken over by exhaustion, or I don't feel like doing more self-care. I just want to not have to do it anymore. I want to not have to do all this stuff just to function. Then I remember that some things have really helped me, like exercise, supplements, and therapy. I feel calmer, and most days I have enough energy. Many days I have less pain, but I may never be completely pain-free. Even with this, I will keep going. Because I want to lead a full life, even with a long illness. I hope this is not my forever, but it might be. I'm not getting a different body, a different nervous system. So I'm continuing on. My life is filled with so many good things. And I already have proof that some things help, and that's made a big difference.

It feels hard to end a book about long illness when long illness itself rarely has a clear one. In writing this book, we kept adding chapters, adding tools, and adding stories. We still do not feel that we have reached the end. The journey will continue. What we do know is that there is so much more to be learned about long illness. We are in need of well-designed research, targeted therapeutics, and greater public awareness.

Long illness follows no consistent pattern. For some, long illness will last a few months and resolve. For many, some symptoms will improve while others persist. Others experience periods of well-being followed by seemingly endless struggle. And then there are illnesses that worsen, despite all our best efforts. At every turn, we hope this book can join you and offer tools and support.

Turn to a story that resonated with you in moments of isolation. Use the journaling prompts to help you when you are feeling stuck. Pick up our tools and exercises to help you find your center in the storm of a particularly bad day of long illness.

If a new symptom comes up, refer to a chapter you may have only skimmed before. See what resonates for you. Underline, circle, and fill out the exercises. Try new tools, journal, and listen for an intuitive sense of what your body needs.

Use this book as a jumping-off point to advocate for your own health care. Take it with you to medical appointments. Let it educate a busy practitioner who may not have expertise in long illness or lacks exposure to integrative approaches. You deserve more. This book can help.

For example, you could bring the headache chapter to your primary practitioner to discuss your headaches. This may help you to push for a referral to a specialized headache neurologist. With this book, you can feel like we are in the room with you, saying, "Try something else, listen to what they are saying, consider an integrative therapy."

It is said that change is the only constant. But in a long illness, some things don't change, or they don't change on the time line we want or need. It can be useful to focus on the aspects of managing a long illness that can change. In our practice, we go back to the basics: a health-promoting diet to reduce inflammation and the risk of numerous diseases; moving the body in order to reduce inflammation, pain, and fatigue; a mindfulness practice to shift the nervous system, which can affect nearly every organ; and tools for psychological growth, which can impact the body and change your experience of the world. Refer to our chapters on each of these strategies for help in making small but mighty changes.

Your suffering should be met with compassionate care. We know that this doesn't happen enough. In our introduction, we mentioned the concept of social determinants of health, which may play a role in your life, impacting your ability to get the health care you need. Healing is more likely to occur within safe, secure relationships. With long illness, such relationships can be harder to find, even as they are more essential than ever. In our clinics, relationships can last years. We like it that way. This book reflects our philosophy of healing: personalized, evidence-based integrative care in a supportive space.

Our hope is that our connection with you is just beginning. We will continue to share tools and important updates. We hope to hear your stories and experiences as well.

Healing doesn't always take place along a straight path. Healing can be occurring even in the midst of suffering. There is inevitably pain in life, especially with long illness. It worsens with loneliness, and when it is repressed or shamed. Make space for your suffering. Use this book to both acknowledge your experiences and find mindful tools to lighten the load. And on days when you feel better, allow for that too.

And continue to breathe.

EXERCISE

END AND CONTINUE ON

Join us in a final mindfulness exercise to reflect on your experience with the book.

Find a quiet space. Follow along on audio or read this script.

Take a moment to center yourself. Take long, slow, deep breaths.

Keep breathing. Read or listen to the following statements. They encapsulate how we feel about you and what we hope for your recovery moving forward. Allow these statements to wash over you. Reflect on their meaning. Hold on to the statements that ring true for you, pause on those that feel out of reach, and honor any part of yourself that still doesn't feel that what they claim is possible.

There are people like me. I am not alone.

There are people who can help me. I am not abandoned.

My body has the capacity to shift. Change is a constant.

I have knowledge and tools.

I am part of a global movement.
I am seen.
I can persist.

We walk beside you, wherever you are.

Warmly,
Dr. Morgan and Dr. Jobson

Appendix A

Personal Health Log

	Name, Contact Info, Notes
Your Medical Team	
The Basics	
Insurance	
Pharmacy	
Primary Practitioner	
Emergency Contact	
Medical Decision-Maker	
Other Practitioners	

	Name, Contact Info, Notes	Last Visited? Next Visit?
Therapist		
Dentist		
Vision Care		
Physical Therapy/ Occupational Therapy		
Specialist		

Specialist		
Specialist		
Other		
Other		
Other		

Appendix B

Activity Log

Goal: Keep an activity log for one week.

	Example	MONDAY	TUESDAY	WEDNESDAY	THURSDAY	FRIDAY	SATURDAY	SUNDAY
12:00–1:00 a.m.	Sleep							
1:00–2:00 a.m.	Sleep							
2:00–3:00 a.m.	Sleep							
3:00–4:00 a.m.	Sleep							
4:00–5:00 a.m.	Up, walked 5 minutes							
5:00–6:00 a.m.	Sleep							
6:00–7:00 a.m.	Read in bed							
7:00–8:00 a.m.	Made food 10 minutes							
8:00–9:00 a.m.	5-minute walk							
9:00–10:00 a.m.	In bed							
10:00–11:00 a.m.	Nap							
11:00–12:00 p.m.	Nap							
12:00–1:00 p.m.	Made lunch							
1:00–2:00 p.m.	20-minute walk							
2:00–3:00 p.m.	Sat outside							
3:00–4:00 p.m.	Laundry 5 minutes							
4:00–5:00 p.m.	5-minute dog walk							
5:00–6:00 p.m.	Made dinner 20 minutes							
6:00–7:00 p.m.	Washed dishes 5 minutes							
7:00–8:00 p.m.	PT exercises 5 minutes							
8:00–9:00 p.m.	Sleep							
9:00–10:00 p.m.	Awake, TV							
10:00–11:00 p.m.	TV							
11:00–12:00 p.m.	TV							
Activity minutes	80 minutes							

Appendix C

Sleep Log

Date	Time I Got into Bed	Time I Fell Asleep	Awakenings (Number, Duration)	Wake-up Time	Total Sleep Time	Quality of Sleep	Naps (Number, Duration)	Notes About the Day
July 12	9:00 p.m.	10:30 p.m.	1 awakening 1 hour	6:15 a.m.	6 hours, 45 minutes	Good	1 at 12:00 p.m. 30 minutes	Mild back pain, 2 glasses of wine with dinner
July 13	10:00 p.m.	11:30 p.m.	2 awakenings (3 minutes each)	6:30 a.m.	6 hours	Poor	1 at 2:00 p.m. 90 minutes	High stress level, brain fog

Appendix D

Headache Log

Date	Time (Start and End Time, Duration)	Triggers	Severity (10 = Worst Pain, 0 = No Pain)	Symptoms	Treatment Used	Relief (None, Some, Complete)

Appendix E

Micronutrients, Macronutrients, and Trace Minerals

Water-Soluble Vitamins	Functions	Foods
Choline (similar to B vitamins, but not a true vitamin)	Energy metabolism, liver health Memory and brain health Muscle control	Egg yolks, soy, fish, broccoli, liver
Thiamine (B_1)	Energy metabolism Supports nervous system	Yeast, legumes, bananas, nuts, liver, whole-grain bread
Riboflavin (B_2)	Energy metabolism Supports eyes, skin, and nervous system	Green vegetables, yeast, milk, eggs, fish, meats, mushrooms
Niacin (B_3)	Energy metabolism Supports nervous system, skin, and gut health	Eggs, wheat, fish, meats
Pantothenic acid (B_5)	Energy metabolism	Egg yolks, broccoli, kidney, milk, avocados, mushrooms
Pyridoxine (B_6)	Energy metabolism Immune function Regulates hormones Makes neurotransmitters, heme, fats in the brain	Vegetables, bananas, oats, fish, nuts, whole grains, meats
Biotin (B_7)	Helps make amino acids and fatty acids Made in the bowel	Very low levels in food; body usually makes enough without needing it from diet (*Note*: Can interfere with some lab tests)
Folate (B_9)	Makes DNA and RNA Makes healthy red blood cells Helps cells divide	Vegetables, legumes, liver, fortified cereals
Cobalamin (B_{12})	Energy metabolism Makes DNA and RNA Keeps nerves and blood cells healthy Makes red blood cells	Meats, fish, milk, cheese, eggs, fortified cereals, seaweed
Ascorbic acid (C)	Wound healing Collagen synthesis Antioxidant Makes skin healthy Supports blood vessels and bones Protects and maintains cells	Citrus fruits, peppers, kiwi, potatoes

Fat-Soluble Vitamins	Functions	Foods
Vitamin A	Supports immune system, vision, and reproduction Skin and bone health	Retinol: cheese, eggs, oily fish, dairy, liver Beta-carotene: yellow, green, and red vegetables, including leafy greens, yellow fruits like mango
Vitamin D	Bone, teeth, and muscle health Regulates calcium and phosphate Supports immune system	Sun Oily fish, red meat, liver, egg yolks, mushrooms (Note: Vitamin D is added to some foods)
Vitamin E	Antioxidant in metabolism Supports skin and eye health Supports immune system health	Nuts, seeds, olive oil, leafy greens
Vitamin K	Blood clotting Wound healing Makes bones and tissues healthy	Leafy green vegetables, vegetable oils, cereal grains

Macro Minerals	Functions	Foods
Calcium	Bone health Blood clotting Neurotransmission Muscle contraction	Kale, dairy, sardines, salmon, soy, fortified products
Chloride	Fluid balance Control of stomach acid	Seaweed, tomatoes, olives, celery, rye
Magnesium	Muscle contraction Makes proteins Neurotransmission	Pumpkin seeds, chia seeds, almonds, spinach, soy milk
Phosphorus	Bone health Blood pH	Milk, soy, beans, lentils, nuts, whole grains
Potassium	Fluid balance Muscle contraction Neurotransmission	Greens, avocados, salmon, bananas, potatoes, tomatoes
Sodium	Fluid balance Muscle contraction Neurotransmission	Milk, cheese, processed foods, seafood, eggs
Sulfur	Makes protein	Eggs, sesame seeds, cheese, Brazil nuts, soy

Trace Minerals	Functions	Foods
Chromium	Needed for insulin to function	Lettuce, grape juice, whole-wheat bread, brewer's yeast, green beans
Copper	Helps iron and enzymes function	Oysters, shiitake mushrooms, tofu, sweet potatoes, dark chocolate, avocados
Fluoride	Healthy teeth and bones	Spinach, grapes, potatoes, black tea, city water
Iodine	Makes thyroid hormone Supports growth and metabolism	Seaweed, seafood, iodized salt, dairy products
Iron	Carries oxygen Helps make energy	Mussels, sardines, tofu, beans, apricots, pumpkin seeds, raisins, broccoli, poultry
Manganese	Supports enzyme function	Whole grains, legumes, nuts, seafood, leafy vegetables, pepper
Molybdenum	Supports enzyme function	Legumes, whole grains, nuts
Selenium	Antioxidant	Brazil nuts, seafood, brown rice
Zinc	Supports immune system Helps with wound healing Needed for growth Makes proteins and DNA	Seafood, tofu, poultry, hemp seeds, lentils, oatmeal, shiitake mushrooms

Appendix F

Your Life Tree

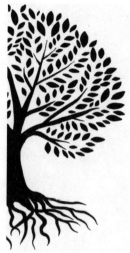

Leaves What does your life look like today?
Important people, hobbies, career, hopes, dreams

Branches What roles or experiences helped define you?
 Big events, life roles

Trunk Who did you grow into?
Skills, abilities, talents, values

Roots Where do you come from?
Family, culture, childhood experiences and hobbies

Resources

Here are apps, books, podcasts, websites, and workbooks that our communities have found helpful. We look forward to learning about what has worked for you so that we can grow our list.

ADHD

The Adult ADHD Tool Kit: Using CBT to Facilitate Coping Inside and Out by J. Russell Ramsay and Anthony L. Rostain

Children and Adults with Attention Deficit Hyperactivity Disorder, CHADD.org, https://chadd.org/diversity/: Education, advocacy, and support groups for ADHD

The Smart but Scattered Guide to Success: How to Use Your Brain's Executive Skills to Keep Up, Stay Calm, and Get Organized at Work and at Home by Peg Dawson and Richard Guare

Thriving with Adult ADHD: Skills to Strengthen Executive Functioning by Phil Boissiere

Detox

Environmental Working Group, https://www.ewg.org

Diet and Nutrition

The Appetite Awareness Workbook: How to Listen to Your Body and Overcome Bingeing, Overeating, and Obsession with Food by Linda W. Craighead

Center for Mindful Eating, www.thecenterformindfuleating.org

Decolonizing Wellness: A QTBIPOC-Centered Guide to Escape the Diet Trap, Heal Your Self-Image, and Achieve Body Liberation by Dalia Kinsey

Eat Yourself Healthy by Megan Rossi

Environmental Working Group, "Good Food on a Tight Budget," www
.ewg.org/goodfood

Feeding America, www.feedingamerica.org: Food bank information

Monash University, "The Low FODMAP Diet," www.monashfodmap.com

MySymptoms food diary app, www.mysymptoms.net

Dysautonomia

Dysautonomic Information Network, www.dinet.org

Dysautonomic International, www.dysautonomiainternational.org

General Mental Health Resources

*The Mindfulness Workbook for OCD: A Guide to Overcoming Obsessions and
Compulsions Using Mindfulness and Cognitive Behavioral Therapy* by Jon
Hershfield

NAMI, Your Journey, www.nami.org/Your-Journey/Individuals-with
-Mental-Illness: Provides information on identity and cultural dimensions of mental illness

Set Boundaries, Find Peace: A Guide to Reclaiming Yourself by Nedra Glover
Tawwab

This Too Shall Pass: Stories of Change, Crisis, and Hopeful Beginnings by Julia
Samuel

*The Unapologetic Guide to Black Mental Health: Navigate an Unequal Sys-
tem, Learn Tools for Emotional Wellness, and Get the Help You Deserve* by
Rheeda Walker

*We've Been Too Patient: Voices from Radical Mental Health—Stories and
Research Challenging the Biomedical Model* by L. D. Green and Kelechi
Ubozoh

Headaches

American Migraine Foundation, https://americanmigrainefoundation
.org/

Splitting: The Inside Story on Headaches by Amanda Ellison

Illness, Identity, Self-Advocacy, Disability Awareness, Community, and Team Building

Belong: Find Your People, Create Community, and Live a More Connected Life by Radha Agrawal

Black Disability Politics by Sami Schalk

A Burst of Light and Other Essays by Audre Lorde

Care Work: Dreaming Disability Justice by Leah Lakshmi Piepzna-Samarasinha

The Collected Schizophrenias: Essays by Esmé Weijun Wang

Disability Visibility: First-Person Stories from the Twenty-First Century, edited by Alice Wong

Easy Beauty: A Memoir by Chloé Cooper Jones

Family Caregiver Alliance, www.caregiver.org

GoodRx, www.goodrx.com: Offers discounts on brand-name and generic medications

Health in Her Hue, https://healthinherhue.com: Connects Black women and women of color to culturally sensitive health care providers, evidence-based health content, and community support

Invisible: How Young Women with Serious Health Issues Navigate Work, Relationships, and the Pressure to Seem Just Fine by Michele Lent Hirsch

The Invisible Kingdom: Reimagining Chronic Illness by Meghan O'Rourke

The Isolation Journals, www.theisolationjournals.com: Free weekly journaling prompts to fuel creativity and encourage community

On Being Ill by Virginia Woolf

What Doesn't Kill You: A Life with Chronic Illness—Lessons from a Body in Revolt by Tessa Miller

Year of the Tiger: An Activist's Life by Alice Wong

Mental Health Crisis Line (Includes Spanish and Other Languages Upon Request)

988 Suicide and Crisis Lifeline, 988, https://988lifeline.org/

Mindfulness, Meditation, Deep Breathing, and Biofeedback

Association for Applied Psychophysiology and Biofeedback, www.aapb.org

Calm app: An introduction to mindfulness with instructions, a guided body scan, relaxation scenes, and sounds to support self-guided meditation

Free guided meditations: Search online for "free guided meditation," as well as for Jon Kabat-Zinn, Tara Brach, Kristen Neff, Marty Rossman, Jack Kornfield

Headspace app: Teaches the basics of meditation and mindfulness in just ten minutes per day

HeartMath, www.heartmath.com

Kardia app: A hands-on, paced breathing exercise

The Little Book of Being: Practices and Guidance for Uncovering Your Natural Awareness by Diana Winston

Mindfulness by Ellen J. Langer

Mindfulness for Beginners: Reclaiming the Present Moment—and Your Life and other books by Jon Kabat-Zinn

A Mindfulness-Based Stress Reduction Workbook by Bob Stahl and Elisha Goldstein

The Miracle of Mindfulness: An Introduction to the Practice of Meditation by Thich Nhat Hanh

Palouse Mindfulness: Mindfulness-Based Stress Reduction, http://palousemindfulness.com/selfguidedMBSR.html: Free online instruction, in multiple languages

Self-Compassion: The Proven Power of Being Kind to Yourself by Kristin Neff

Unf*ck Your Brain: Getting Over Anxiety, Depression, Anger, Freak-Outs, and Triggers . . . with Science! by Faith Harper

Pain

An Anatomy of Pain: How the Body and the Mind Experience and Endure Physical Suffering by Abdul-Ghaaliq Lalkhen

FibroGuide, https://fibroguide.med.umich.edu: An online symptom management program for people living with fibromyalgia

Full Catastrophe Living: Using the Wisdom of Your Body and Mind to Face Stress, Pain, and Illness by Jon Kabat-Zinn

The Graded Motor Imagery Handbook by David S. Butler, G. Lorimer Moseley, Timothy B. Beames, and Thomas J. Giles

Managing Chronic Pain: A Cognitive-Behavioral Therapy Approach Workbook by John D. Otis

National Fibromyalgia and Chronic Pain Association, www.fmaware .org: Support groups and education

Pain Woman Takes Your Keys, and Other Essays from a Nervous System by Sonya Huber

PTSD Coach, https://mobile.va.gov/app/ptsd-coach: Assists individuals with chronic pain who experienced trauma to learn about, track, and manage symptoms

The Song of Our Scars: The Untold Story of Pain by Haider Warraich

Stanford Model/Chronic Pain Self-Management Program, http:// www.eblcprograms.org/evidence-based/recommended-programs /chronic-pain-self-management/: A community-based intervention delivered once a week for six weeks. Usually free or low-cost to participate. Group sessions last six weeks with two hours of group sessions per week.

You Are Not Your Pain: Using Mindfulness to Relieve Pain, Reduce Stress, and Restore Well-Being—An Eight-Week Program by Vidyamala Burch and Danny Penman

Psychedelic Clinical Trial Databases

Multidisciplinary Association for Psychedelic Studies (MAPS), https:// maps.org/take-action/participate-in-trial

Psychedelic Support, https://psychedelic.support/resources/how-to-join -psychedelic-clinical-trial

Sleep Disturbances and Insomnia

CBT-i Coach App, https://mobile.va.gov/app/cbt-i-coach

The Insomnia Workbook: A Comprehensive Guide to Getting the Sleep You Need by Stephanie Silberman

Quiet Your Mind and Get to Sleep: Solutions to Insomnia for Those with Depression, Anxiety, or Chronic Pain by Colleen Carney and Rachel Manber

Sleep Wise: How to Feel Better, Work Smarter, and Build Resilience by Daniel Blum

Sleepio, Sleepio.com: Six-week sleep improvement program based in CBT; the cost could be cheaper than therapy copays, and the program can be done at home when you have time

Why We Sleep: Unlocking the Power of Sleep and Dreams by Matthew Walker

Support Groups

Friendship Line, www.ioaging.org/services/friendship-line: Toll-free friendship line providing noncrisis peer support for people ages sixty and older and for adults living with disabilities

National Alliance on Mental Illness, https://nami.org/Support-Education/Support-Groups

SAMHSA's National Helpline, 1-800-662-HELP (4357) (also known as the Treatment Referral Routing Service), or TTY: 1-800-487-4889: A confidential, free, 24-hour-per-day, 365-day-per-year information service, in English and Spanish, for individuals and family members facing mental and/or substance use disorders. This service provides referrals to local treatment facilities, support groups, and community-based organizations.

Talley, www.talleyapp.com: A confidential and anonymous place to be heard and accepted

Therapy

The Anxiety and Phobia Workbook by Edmund J. Bourne (CBT)

Ayana Therapy, www.ayanatherapy.com: Mental health care for marginalized and intersectional communities

The Dialectical Behavior Therapy Skills Workbook: Practical DBT Exercises for Learning Mindfulness, Interpersonal Effectiveness, Emotion Regulation, and Distress Tolerance by Matthew McKay, Jeffrey C. Wood, and Jeffrey Brantley

Feeling Good: The New Mood Therapy by David D. Burns (CBT)

I'm Working on It in Therapy: How to Get the Most Out of Psychotherapy by Gary Trosclair

Internal Family Systems: Skills Training Manual: Trauma-Informed Treatment for Anxiety, Depression, PTSD, and Substance Abuse by Frank G. Anderson, Martha Sweezy, and Richard C. Schwartz

Maybe You Should Talk to Someone: A Therapist, Her Therapist, and Our Lives Revealed by Lori Gottlieb

Melanin and Mental Health, www.melaninandmentalhealth.com: *Between Sessions* (podcast)

Self-Therapy Workbook: An Exercise Book for the IFS Process by Bonnie J. Weiss

Shine, www.theshineapp.com: A daily mental wellness app

Therapy for Black Girls, https://therapyforblackgirls.com

The Worry Trap: How to Free Yourself from Worry and Anxiety Using Acceptance and Commitment Therapy by Chad LeJeune (ACT)

The Yoga Effect: A Proven Program for Depression and Anxiety by Liz Owen and Holly Lebowitz Rossi

Traditional Medicine, Supplements, and Natural Products

National Ayurvedic Medical Association, www.ayurvedanama.org

National Certification Commission for Acupuncture and Oriental Medicine, www.nccaom.org/find-a-practitioner-directory

Natural Medicine Database, https://naturalmedicines.therapeutic research.com

People's Organization of Community Acupuncture, www.pocacoop .com: Community acupuncture, sliding scale, and low-fee

Trauma

The Body Keeps the Score: Brain, Mind, and Body in the Healing of Trauma by Bessel van der Kolk

Life After Trauma: A Workbook for Healing by Dena Rosenbloom and Mary Beth Williams

My Grandmother's Hands: Racialized Trauma and the Pathway to Mending Our Hearts and Bodies by Resmaa Menakem

The Myth of Normal: Trauma, Illness, and Healing in a Toxic Culture by Gabor Maté and Daniel Maté

Transcending Trauma: Healing Complex PTSD with Internal Family Systems Therapy by Frank Anderson

What Happened to You? Conversations on Trauma, Resilience, and Healing by Oprah Winfrey and Bruce D. Perry

What My Bones Know: A Memoir of Healing from Complex Trauma by Stephanie Foo

References

Available upon request

Acknowledgments

Our deepest gratitude to:

The patients, health care workers, educators, researchers, and advocates who inspire us to be better humans and stronger practitioners. You provided us with the knowledge to write this book.

Laura Yorke, our agent, who helped us find an outlet for our passion.

Renee Sedliar, our editor, for caring so deeply about this project.

Katy Sims and Hannah L. Kirsch, for editorial support; you helped us find our voice.

Our sharp-eyed readers who offered generous feedback: Elizabeth Abbs, Jennifer Ashby, Theora Cimino, Rita Crooms, Niki Flacks, Joel Horovitz, Brendan Huang, Lina Khouer, Julian Motzkin, Tianyi Zhang, Kristin Nguyen, Morgan Stewart, and Ben Wolinsky.

The Hachette Go team, including Michelle Aielli, Michael Barrs, Alison Dalafave, Quinn Fariel, Kindall Gant, Mike Giarratano, Sean Moreau, Mary Ann Naples, and Terri Sirma.

Our UCSF mentors and community, including Brieze Bell, John Chamberlain, Caitlin Costello, Anand Dhruva, Erick Hung, S. Andrew Josephson, Carla Kuon, Michael Levin, Lekshmi Santhosh, and Kathy Waller.

Gabrielle deFiebre, James Duffy, Veronica Jacobs, Heather Jones, Lizzie Jones, Sara LaHue, Heidi Montague, Dave Owen, Julie Rehmeyer, Lindsey Ryan, Olivia Spring, Maria Germaine Vogel, and Kristen Winsor, for their perspectives and insights into long illness.

Our supportive families, friends, and communities. We have learned so much from you. This book would not exist without you.

Notes

1. Joseph Conrad, *Lord Jim* (London: Oxford University Press, 1982).
2. US Department of Justice, Civil Rights Division, "A Guide to Disability Rights Laws," February 2020, www.ada.gov/cguide.htm.
3. Social Security Administration, "Access to Employment Support Services for Social Security Disability Beneficiaries Who Want to Work," choosework.ssa.gov. Many other countries offer similar programs to encourage people who are disabled and want to work to do so. Navigating the US program can be complicated, but members of your care team can help you.
4. *Opioids* are all-natural, synthetic, and semisynthetic opioids. *Opiates* are the natural opioids only (heroin, morphine, codeine). You might hear both terms being used.
5. For example, see GetNaloxoneNow at www.getnaloxonenow.org/#home and NEXT Distro at nextdistro.org/naloxone#state-finder.
6. We provide these numbers as an example of the type of information you can get out of a food diary. For many people, knowing calorie and nutrient density is helpful in better understanding the quality of their diet. For others, it can feel irrelevant or even shaming. If the latter is your experience, skip over these numbers. You can reflect on a food diary and eat in health-promoting ways without worrying about calories or grams of fat. Don't calculate nutrients unless knowing these numbers is helpful in moving you toward vitality.
7. US Department of Agriculture, "Healthy Eating on a Budget," www.myplate.gov /eat-healthy/healthy-eating-budget. Nutrition and diet research is complicated and fraught with controversy. The USDA "Dietary Guidelines for Americans," which shape the nutritional contents of prison, military, and school lunches, are referenced throughout this chapter. However, the USDA guidelines leave a lot to be desired. For example, despite evidence, they are too lenient concerning the ingestion of sodas, sugary drinks, and sugar-laden foods, as well as with regard to decreasing alcohol and avoiding red and processed meat, and they overemphasize the importance of dairy. Our reading of the data makes this clear: sugar, saturated fats, salt, and alcohol are overwhelmingly not good for you in the amounts they are usually consumed, and even at low levels they can be pro-inflammatory. Nevertheless, the USDA guidelines provide a great way to start thinking more about your diet and how to improve it.

8. National Heart, Lung, and Blood Institute, "DASH Eating Plan," www.nhlbi.nih.gov /health-topics/dash-eating-plan (last updated December 29, 2021).

9. As we discussed earlier, *ableism* is characterizing people with an illness or disability as less capable or whole than someone who is not ill or disabled.

10. Some physical therapists or sports medicine practitioners offer a technique called *dry needling*, which is not acupuncture and should not be confused with it. Dry needling is used to help with injuries, muscle pain, and fibromyalgia. There is minimal evidence for the effectiveness of this practice, and it is unregulated. If it helps you feel better, however, and it is within your budget, enjoy.

11. Auricular acupuncture is used on the battlefield and for addiction detox with the National Acupuncture Detoxification Association protocol.

12. Go to the website of the People's Organization of Community Acupuncture (www .pocacoop.com/places) to see if there is a community clinic near you.

13. See the Natural Medicines Comprehensive Database: Consumer Version (naturaldata baseconsumer.therapeuticresearch.com). A more comprehensive version is available for practitioners.

Index